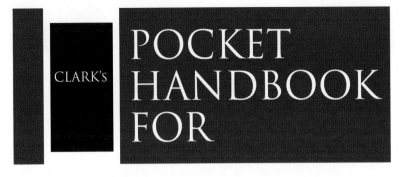

POCKET HANDBOOK FOR

CLARK'S

RADIOGRAPHERS

T0144502

Drawn from the renowned reference *Clark's Positioning in Radiography*, this bestselling pocket handbook provides clear and practical advice to help radiographers in their day-to-day work. Designed and structured for rapid reference, it covers how to position the patient and image receptor as well as the direction and location of the beam, describes the essential image characteristics, and illustrates each radiographic projection with a positioning photograph and corresponding radiographic image.

This third edition has been updated to include new positioning photographs reflecting the dominance of direct digital radiography detectors (DDRs), helpful information on the importance of optimisation, exposure factors and geometry in image production, evaluating exposure in digital imaging and aspects of bariatric imaging.

Clark's Companion Essential Guides

Series Editor
A Stewart Whitley

Clark's Essential PACS, RIS and Imaging Informatics
Alexander Peck

Clark's Essential Physics in Imaging for Radiographers, 2E
Ken Holmes, Marcus Elkington, Phil Harris

Clark's Essential Guide to Clinical Ultrasound
Jan Dodgeon, Gill Harrison

Clark's Essential Guide to Mammography
Claire Borrelli, Claire Mercer

Clark's Pocket Handbook for Radiographers, 3E
A Stewart Whitley, Charles Sloane, Gail Jefferson, Ken Holmes, Craig Anderson

https://www.routledge.com/Clarks-Companion-Essential-Guides/book-series/CRCCLACOMESS

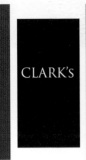

CLARK'S

POCKET HANDBOOK FOR

RADIOGRAPHERS

THIRD EDITION

A Stewart Whitley, Radiology Advisor, UK Radiology Advisory Services, Preston, Lancashire, UK and Former Director of Professional Practice, International Society of Radiographers and Radiological Technologists (ISRRT)

Charles Sloane, Principal Lecturer and Professional Lead for Health Sciences, Institute of Health, University of Cumbria, Lancaster, UK

Gail Jefferson, Senior Lecturer and Programme Lead for Diagnostic Radiography, Institute of Health, University of Cumbria, Lancaster; Reporting Radiographer, North Cumbria Integrated Care, Carlisle, UK

Ken Holmes, formerly Senior Lecturer, Institute of Health, University of Cumbria, Lancaster, UK

Craig Anderson, Senior Lecturer, Institute of Health, University of Cumbria, Lancaster; Clinical Tutor and Reporting Radiographer, Furness General Hospital, Cumbria, UK

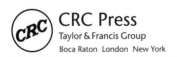

CRC Press
Taylor & Francis Group
Boca Raton London New York

CRC Press is an imprint of the
Taylor & Francis Group, an **informa** business

Designed cover image: Shutterstock image - 228726352[9]

Third edition published 2024
by CRC Press
2385 NW Executive Center Drive, Suite 320, Boca Raton, FL 33431

and by CRC Press
4 Park Square, Milton Park, Abingdon, Oxon, OX14 4RN

CRC Press is an imprint of Taylor & Francis Group, LLC

© 2024 A Stewart Whitley, Charles Sloane, Gail Jefferson, Ken Holmes and Craig Anderson

First Edition published – 2010
Second Edition published – 2017

ISBN: 978-1-032-04338-8 (hbk)
ISBN: 978-1-032-04337-1 (pbk)
ISBN: 978-1-003-19152-0 (ebk)

DOI: 10.1201/ 9781003191520

Typeset in Berling
by Evolution Design & Digital Ltd (Kent)

Printed in Great Britain by Bell and Bain Ltd, Glasgow

CONTENTS

Section 3 Useful Information for Radiographic Practice

PREFACE

This third edition of *Clark's Pocket Handbook for Radiographers* is an accompaniment to the 13th Edition of *Clark's Positioning in Radiography*, a comprehensive bench-top guide to radiographic technique and positioning. The authors considered that it is important for radiographers and students to have access to an additional text available in a 'pocket' format which is easily transportable and convenient to use during everyday radiographic practice.

While it has been impossible to include all the radiographic projections from the 13th Edition due to size restrictions, the authors have included what they consider to be the most commonly used projections. Readers are advised to consult the 13th Edition of *Clark's Positioning in Radiography* if they seek guidance in undertaking any projections that have not been included in this book.

As the book evolves it reflects those changes and challenges that are now common in many imaging departments, especially with the widespread use of digital imaging in the form of direct digital radiography (DDR) detectors, whether portable or fixed. This is in contrast to computed radiography (CR) technology which is now on the decline, with a variety of different CR cassette sizes to match the area of interest.

Additionally, it is important for the reader to understand fundamentally the relationship of dose and image quality in the digital environment. We have added several new materials relating to the importance of optimisation and exposure factors, evaluating exposure and digital imaging, as well as bariatric imaging.

The various projections described in this book have been produced from the 13th Edition of *Clark's Positioning in Radiography*. The main changes to the first and second editions are outlined below.

The title 'Direction and Centring of the X-ray Beam' has been changed to 'Direction and Location of the X-ray Beam' to remind students of the importance to collimate and position the beam to include the specific area of interest as well as considering the centring point.

UK national and local diagnostic reference levels (DRLs) have been added to most X-ray examinations as a reminder of the importance of optimisation and keeping a record of patient doses. Readers should be aware of their local DRLs.

Readers should also be aware of the recent national and international advice on the routine use of gonad shielding, which was taken into account when updating the second edition of the *Handbook*.

A section on basic skull CT examination has been added to reflect the comprehensive role of the radiographer.

Unless otherwise stated, the standard focus-to-receptor distance (FRD) for all examinations described is 100 cm for direct/extremity work and 110 cm for Bucky/table work. Note that, in the book, whereas we use the term vertical Bucky, it can also be referred to as a wall Bucky stand, a wall Bucky unit or a radiographic wall stand.

Finally, students and readers are directed to Section 3 where they will find both valuable and useful information for radiographic practice with details of non-diagnostic tests and explanations of medical terminology and medical and radiographic abbreviations.

ACKNOWLEDGEMENTS

The authors would like to acknowledge the work of all the authors and the models, mostly students from the University of Cumbria, who posed for the photographs for this third edition, plus those who modelled for the 13th Edition of *Clark's Positioning in Radiography* and previous editions.

The book is inspired by the original work and dedication of Kathleen C Clark and subsequent authors of the *Clark's Positioning in Radiography* series of textbooks whose objective was to produce a meaningful and descriptive text for a new generation of radiographers.

Our thanks go to Joshua Holmes and Stewart Whitley who ably undertook a number of new positioning photographs and Dr Amanda Martin, Radiography Consultant, UK, who provided advice on a number of aspects of positioning technique.

We would like to thank colleagues who provided images to accompany the positioning photos and Dr Stephen Fenn, Hampshire Hospitals NHS Foundation Trust, who kindly provided the prone chest X-ray image.

Mention must also be given to Paul Charnock, Radiation Protection Advisor, and Ben Thomas, Technical Officer, both from Integrated Radiological Services (IRS) Ltd, Liverpool, UK, who provided examples of local diagnostic reference levels.

SECTION 1
KEY ASPECTS OF RADIOGRAPHIC PRACTICE

ANATOMICAL TERMINOLOGY

The human body is a complicated structure. Errors in radiographic positioning or diagnosis can easily occur unless practitioners have a common set of rules that are used to describe the body and its movements. All the basic terminology descriptions below refer to the patient in the standard reference position, known as the anatomical position.

Patient Aspect (Figs. 1.1a–e)

- Anterior aspect is that seen when viewing the patient from the front.
- Posterior (dorsal) aspect is that seen when viewing the patient from the back.
- Lateral aspect refers to any view of the patient from the side. The side of the head would therefore be the lateral aspect of the cranium.
- Medial aspect refers to the side of a body part closest to the midline, e.g. the inner side of a limb is the medial aspect of that limb.

Planes of the Body (Fig. 1.1f)

Three planes of the body are used extensively for descriptions of positioning both in plain X-ray imaging as well as other cross-sectional imaging techniques. The planes described are mutually at right angles to each other.

- Median sagittal plane (MSP) divides the body into right and left halves.
- Any plane parallel to this but dividing the body into unequal right and left portions, is simply known as a sagittal plane or parasagittal plane.
- Coronal plane divides the body into an anterior part and a posterior part.
- Transverse or axial plane divides the body into a superior part and an inferior part.

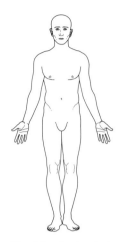

Fig. 1.1a Anatomical position.

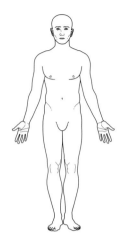

Fig. 1.1b Anterior aspect of body.

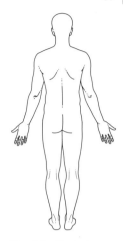

Fig. 1.1c Posterior aspect of body.

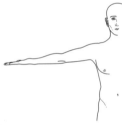

Fig. 1.1d Medial aspect of arm.

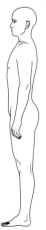

Fig. 1.1e Lateral aspect of body.

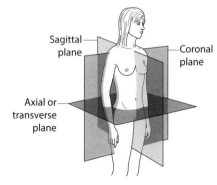

Fig. 1.1f Body planes.

Lines and Landmarks: the Skull (Figs. 1.2a,b)

Landmarks

- Outer canthus of the eye: the point where the upper and lower eyelids meet laterally.
- Infra-orbital margin/point: the lowest point of the inferior rim of the orbit.
- Nasion: the articulation between the nasal and frontal bones.
- Glabella: a bony prominence found on the frontal bone immediately superior to the nasion.
- Vertex: the highest point of the skull in the median sagittal plane.
- External occipital protuberance (inion): a bony prominence found on the occipital bone, usually coincident with the median sagittal plane.
- External auditory meatus (EAM): the opening within the ear that leads into the external auditory canal.

Lines

- Inter-orbital (inter-pupillary) line: joins the centre of the two orbits or the centre of the two pupils when the eyes are looking straight forward.
- Infra-orbital line: joins the two infra-orbital points.
- Anthropological baseline: passes from the infra-orbital point to the upper border of the external auditory meatus (also known as the Frankfort line).
- Orbito-meatal baseline (radiographic baseline): extends from the outer canthus of the eye to the centre of the external auditory meatus. This line is angled approximately 10 degrees to the anthropological baseline.

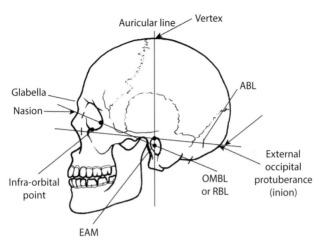

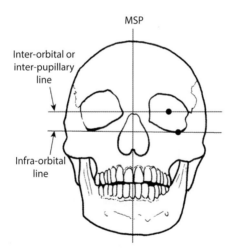

Fig. 1.2a,b Lines and landmarks of the skull.

POSITIONING TERMINOLOGY

This section describes how the patient is positioned for the various radiographic projections described in this text.

Erect: the projection is taken with the patient sitting (Fig. 1.3a) or standing:
- with the posterior aspect against the wall stand/vertical Bucky; or
- with the anterior aspect against the image receptor (Fig. 1.3b); or
- with the right (Fig. 1.3e) or left side against the image receptor.

Decubitus: the patient is lying down. In the decubitus position, the patient may be lying in any of the following positions:
- prone (ventral decubitus): lying face down (Fig. 1.3c);
- supine (dorsal decubitus): lying on their back (Fig. 1.3d);
- lateral decubitus: lying on their side: right lateral decubitus – lying on right side; left lateral decubitus – lying on left side (Fig. 1.3f).

Semi-recumbent: the patient is reclining, part way between supine and sitting erect.

All the positions may be more precisely described by reference to the planes of the body. For example, 'the patient is supine with the MSP at right angles to the table top' or 'the patient is erect with the left side in contact with the image receptor and the coronal plane perpendicular to the image receptor'.

When describing positioning for upper limb projections, the patient will often be 'seated by the table'. Figure 1.3a shows the correct position to be used for upper limb radiography, with the coronal plane approximately perpendicular to the short axis of the table top. The legs will not be under the table, therefore avoiding exposure of the gonads to any primary radiation not attenuated by the image receptor or table.

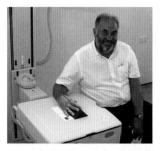

Fig. 1.3a Position for extremity radiography.

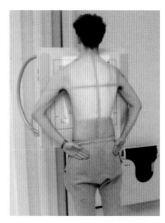

Fig. 1.3b Erect, anterior aspect against the wall stand/vertical Bucky.

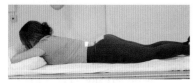

Fig. 1.3c Prone

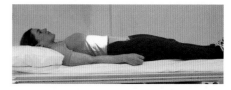

Fig. 1.3d Supine.

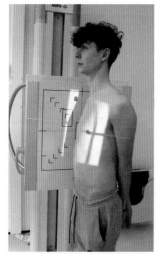

Fig. 1.3e Erect, right side against the wall stand/vertical Bucky.

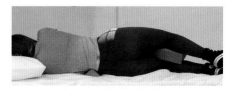

Fig. 1.3f Left lateral decubitus.

Terminology Used to Describe the Limb Positions (Figs. 1.4a–h)

Positioning for limb radiography may include:

- a description of the aspect of the limb in contact with the image receptor;
- the direction of rotation of the limb in relation to the anatomical position, e.g. medial (internal) rotation towards the midline or lateral (external) rotation away from the midline;
- the final angle to the image receptor of a line joining two imaginary landmarks;
- movements and degree of movement of the various joints concerned.

Extension: when the angle of the joint increases.

Flexion: when the angle of the joint decreases.

Abduction: refers to a movement away from the midline.

Adduction: refers to a movement towards the midline.

Rotation: movement of the body part around its own axis, e.g. medial (internal) rotation towards the midline, or lateral (external) rotation away from the midline.

Supination: a movement of the hand and forearm in which the palm is moved from facing posteriorly to anteriorly (as per the anatomical position).

Pronation: the reverse of supination.

Other movement terms applied to specific body parts are described in Figure 1.4.

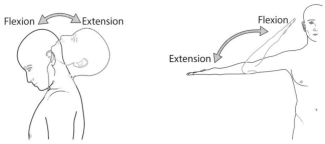

Fig. 1.4a Neck flexion and extension.   **Fig. 1.4b** Elbow flexion and extension.

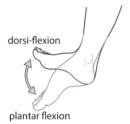

dorsi-flexion

plantar flexion

Fig. 1.4c Foot: dorsi- and plantar flexion.

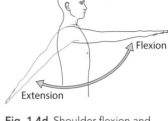

Flexion

Extension

Fig. 1.4d Shoulder flexion and extension.

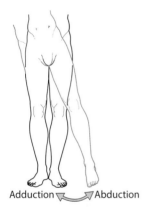

Adduction   Abduction

Fig. 1.4e Hip adduction and abduction.

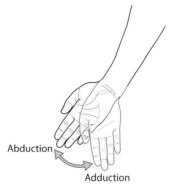

Abduction

Adduction

Fig. 1.4f Wrist adduction and abduction.

Supination

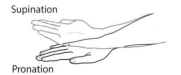

Pronation

Fig. 1.4g Hand pronation and supination.

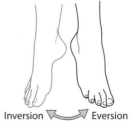

Inversion   Eversion

Fig. 1.4h Foot inversion and eversion.

PROJECTION TERMINOLOGY

A radiographic projection is described by the direction of the central ray relative to aspects and planes of the body.

Antero-posterior (Fig. 1.5a)

The central ray is incident on the anterior aspect, passes along or parallel to the median sagittal plane and emerges from the posterior aspect of the body.

Postero-anterior (Fig. 1.5b)

The central ray is incident on the posterior aspect, passes along or parallel to the median sagittal plane and emerges from the anterior aspect of the body.

Lateral (Fig. 1.5c)

The central ray passes from one side of the body to the other along a coronal and transverse plane. The projection is called a right lateral if the central ray enters the body on the left side and passes through to the image receptor positioned on the right side. A left lateral is achieved if the central ray enters the body on the right side and passes through to an image receptor that is positioned parallel to the MSP on the left side of the body.

In the case of a limb, the central ray is either incident on the lateral aspect and emerges from the medial aspect (latero-medial) or is incident on the medial aspect and emerges from the lateral aspect of the limb (medio-lateral). The terms latero-medial and medio-lateral are used where necessary to differentiate between the two projections.

Beam Angulation

Radiographic projections are often modified by directing the central ray at some angle to a transverse plane, i.e. either caudally (angled towards the feet) or with a cranial/cephalic angulation (angled towards the head). The projection is then described as, for example, a lateral 20-degree caudad or a lateral 15-degree cephalad.

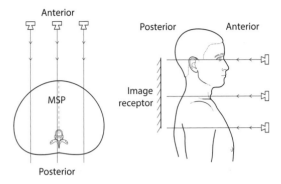

Fig. 1.5a Antero-posterior (AP) projection.

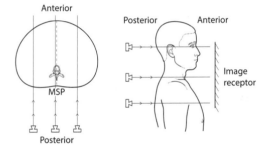

Fig. 1.5b Postero-anterior (PA) projection.

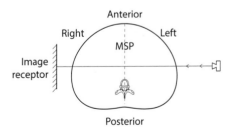

Fig. 1.5c Right lateral projection.

Oblique

The central ray passes through the body along a transverse plane at some angle between the median sagittal and coronal planes. For this projection, the patient is usually positioned with the median sagittal plane at an angle between 0 and 90 degrees to the receptor, with the central ray at right angles to the receptor. If the patient is positioned with the median sagittal plane at right angles to or parallel to the receptor, the projection is obtained by directing the central ray at some angle to the median sagittal plane.

Anterior Oblique (Fig. 1.6a)

The central ray enters the posterior aspect, passes along a transverse plane at some angle to the median sagittal plane and emerges from the anterior aspect. The projection is also described by the side of the torso closest to the receptor. In the figure, the left side is closest to the receptor so the projection is described as a left anterior oblique.

Posterior Oblique (Fig. 1.6b)

The central ray enters the anterior aspect, passes along a transverse plane at some angle to the median sagittal plane and emerges from the posterior aspect. Again the projection is described by the side of the torso closest to the receptor. The figure shows a left posterior oblique.

Oblique Using Beam Angulation (Fig. 1.6c)

When the median sagittal plane is at right angles to the receptor, right and left anterior or posterior oblique projection may be obtained by angling the central ray to the median sagittal plane. NB: This cannot be done if using a grid unless the grid lines are parallel to the central ray.

Lateral Oblique (Fig. 1.6d)

The central ray enters one lateral aspect, passes along a transverse plane at an angle to the coronal plane and emerges from the opposite lateral aspect.

With the coronal plane at right angles to the receptor, lateral oblique projections can also be obtained by angling the central ray to the coronal plane. NB: This cannot be done if using a grid unless the grid lines are parallel to the central ray.

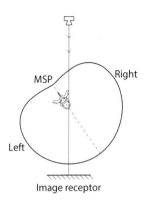

Fig. 1.6a Left anterior oblique projection.

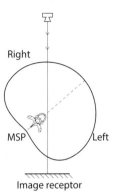

Fig. 1.6b Left posterior oblique projection.

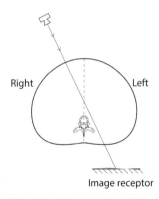

Fig. 1.6c Left posterior oblique obtained using an angled beam.

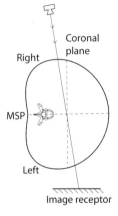

Fig. 1.6d Left lateral oblique projection.

NB: All diagrams are viewed as if looking upwards from the feet.

THE IMPORTANCE OF OPTIMISATION AND EXPOSURE FACTORS

Optimisation of exposure in diagnostic imaging should be built on collaboration between radiologists, radiographers and medical physics experts (MPEs). It should be developed from the initial set up of the X-ray facility and audited to compare with diagnostic reference levels (DRLs) and equipment testing data. Examination parameters and protocols should then be adjusted if necessary, considering image quality. Exposure factors should be established for all anatomical regions and patient characteristics.

Detector dose indicators (DDIs), exposure indices (EIs) and image collimation should also be monitored.

The target exposure index (EI_T) represents the optimal exposure for a particular body part being imaged, patient characteristics and the imaging request. EI_T values should be determined by clinical requirements of the examination and will depend on the minimum noise acceptable.

The use of 0.1–0.3 copper filtration, especially for paediatric exposures, is recommended. This can be used to reduce the effective dose by 20–50% in the 70–80 kV range by removing low-energy photons. The highest kilovoltage within the optimal range for each projection should be used. The lowest tube milliamp-seconds (mAs) is then selected to provide an adequate exposure to the image receptor.

Automatic exposure control (AEC) devices should be employed where they are installed and appropriate to the technique being undertaken. AEC devices should be calibrated to suit the characteristics of each detector and can be set up to maintain a constant EI. The initial setting up of AECs is crucial in determining exposure levels and all chamber combinations should be tested regularly with phantoms representing a range of patient body habitus. To achieve a consistent exposure level, an AEC device is usually employed in fixed radiographic imaging equipment that terminate exposures at predetermined levels. AEC devices have settings that allow the exposure level to be decreased or increased, and these can be used to select lower or higher exposures for particular types of examination.

The central importance of collimation on patient dose and image quality should be emphasised throughout daily clinical practice. Poor collimation irradiates unnecessary adjacent tissue, increasing scatter and patient dose. It can also reduce contrast in the image.

Acceptance testing and commissioning are crucial to ensure new equipment is performing optimally. After commissioning, medical physicists and radiographers should work together to establish a local quality control/quality assurance programme. Radiographers, radiologists, picture archiving and communication system (PACS) managers and medical physicists should collaborate to identify the most appropriate processing algorithms for reporting radiographic images.

Digital radiography has a wide dynamic range which allows for processing of images after exposure. As a result, it is the noise level and image contrast that set the limits on image quality. Selection of tube potential is a compromise between competing requirements, such as contrast and penetration, and appropriate combinations of tube potential and mAs should be established for different anatomical regions and patient characteristics and linked to the clinical question to be answered.

Scattered radiation reduces contrast in radiography and limits the dynamic range of X-ray intensities that is available. Grids are employed to absorb the scattered radiation to improve contrast and are used for the majority of adult radiography examinations of the trunk or head. They are not required when imaging thicknesses of soft tissue less than about 12 cm or for low-attenuation exams with low tube potentials. Grids may be dispensed with for examinations of small children. Modern digital radiography systems may also incorporate virtual grid algorithms where the effect of scatter is digitally corrected in the acquired images. Grids are used with mobile units in which the grids are lighter and easier to handle. Since grids attenuate the transmitted X-ray beam and the specifications vary, exposure factors need to be adjusted upward to maintain the EI. Ideally systems should display an icon to show whether a grid is in place.

Sub-optimal images should be identified through regular audit. Data on rejected images should be collected and analysed on a regular basis. Reject rates should be monitored and calculated so that when they rise above a predetermined threshold action can be taken. Analysing the reasons for rejections should be used to make improvements in working practices.

EVALUATING EXPOSURE IN DIGITAL IMAGING

Modern digital imaging equipment used for projectional radiography has a wide dynamic range. Systems will therefore have a wide exposure latitude. This means that a wide range of exposures (mAs values at a given kV) will produce an image which will appear fit for purpose to the image observer. Grossly underexposed images will look 'grainy' or 'noisy' whereas grossly overexposed images may contain areas of pixel saturation, or black areas in the area of interest. The image may also be generally lacking in contrast.

The wide exposure latitude presents a challenge when assessing the suitability of an exposure for the majority of images that are not grossly under- or overexposed. There is an optimal or 'target' exposure for each body part for each imaging system. This target exposure is determined by the system manufacturer and the system user. It should take into account the DRL for the body part concerned and balance image quality against the dose used to obtain the image.

There are a wide range of exposures above and below this target value which the observer may deem to produce an acceptable image, especially when viewed on a non-reporting monitor. The potential therefore exists to regularly underexpose images that will have a higher level of noise, but this may not be immediately noticeable. Similarly, images which are overexposed may appear to be acceptable but the extra dose of radiation given will not be justified in terms of the small gains in image quality achieved through a reduction in the signal-to-noise ratio.

It is the radiographer's responsibility to ensure that optimal exposure is used at all times. The majority of equipment will possess a DDI which is displayed on the image after an exposure is made. This should be consulted after each exposure to evaluate the success and appropriateness of the exposure factor selection strategy.

Although DDIs can vary between manufacturers, many systems will present three numerical values. The first value is the target exposure index (EI_T). This represents the aforementioned 'ideal exposure'. The second value is the exposure index (EI), a measure of the actual exposure incident on the image detector determined by the exposure factors set by the radiographer.

The final figure is the deviation index (DI) which is a measure of the agreement between the target exposure and the actual exposure incident on the detector. If the image is overexposed, the DI will have a positive value and if underexposed it will have a negative value. A traffic light (Table 1.1) system may also be used which presents the exposure information in a non-numerical way.

Table 1.1 and the associated images present a range of suggested actions should the image evaluation demonstrate a sub-optimal exposure.

Table 1.1 Actions for different DI values.

DI value	Traffic light	Range action
>+3.0 More than double the optimal mAs (Fig. 1.7a)	Red	Excessive exposure: repeat if any anatomy is 'burned out'; requires quality assurance (QA) follow-up and review of set exposure factors.
+1.0 to +3.0 Between 15 and 100% over the optimal mAs (Fig. 1.7b)	Amber	Overexposure: only repeat if anatomy is 'burned out'. If other images of this body part are of a similar value this may require QA follow-up and optimisation of set exposure factors.
−0.5 to +0.5 Up to ±15% of the optimal mAs (Fig. 1.7c)	Green	Target range. No action needed.
<−1.0 to −3.0 Between 15 and 100% under the optimal mAs (Fig. 1.7d)	Amber	Underexposed: review image on a reporting-quality workstation to assess suitability for diagnosis. If this and other images of this body part are of a similar value and are not diagnostic this may require QA follow-up and optimisation of set exposure factors.
<−3.0 Less than half of the optimal mAs (Fig. 1.7e)	Red	Assess noise and suitability for diagnosis; repeat if necessary; requires QA follow-up and review of exposure factors.

NB: Care should be taken when using the 'traffic light' system as the information provided may not always present in a consistent manner. The numerical values are the best method of evaluating the exposure made.

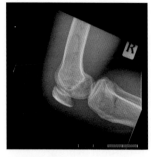

$EI_T = 350$
$EI = 1427$
$DI = 6.1$
60 kV   16 mAs

Fig. 1.7a Grossly overexposed image: note red traffic light. Image is acceptable but not optimal due to overexposure. Needs QA follow-up.

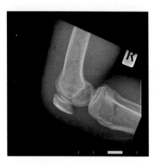

$EI_T = 350$
$EI = 753$
$DI = 3.3$
60 kV   8 mAs

Fig. 1.7b Moderately overexposed image: note yellow traffic light. Image is acceptable but not optimal due to overexposure. Needs QA follow-up.

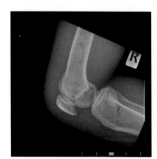

$EI_T = 350$
$EI = 362$
$DI = 0.1$
60 kV   4 mAs

Fig. 1.7c Image exposure within target range: note green traffic light. Exposure optimal.

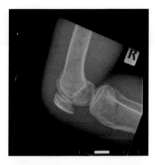

$EI_T = 350$
$EI = 169$
$DI = -3.2$
60 kV   2 mAs

Fig. 1.7d Moderately underexposed image: note yellow traffic light. Image is acceptable but not optimal due to underexposure. Some image noise may be visible on a reporting-quality workstation. Needs QA follow-up.

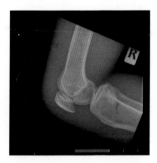

$EI_T = 350$
$EI = 73$
$DI = -6.8$
60 kV   1 mAs

Fig. 1.7e Grossly underexposed image: note red traffic light. Reduced image quality and high noise levels. This will be clearly visible on a reporting-quality workstation and will impact upon the diagnostic potential of the image. The image may need to be repeated and there should be a QA follow-up.

When deciding how to modify the exposure for an image which needs repeating it is worth bearing in mind the following 'rule of thumb'. A DI value of 3 above or below the target value represents an overexposure of double or half of the optimal value. The mAs should therefore be doubled or halved to compensate. *Do not alter the kV when correcting exposure factors as the DDI will not then behave in a consistent manner.*

When considering the underexposed image in Fig. 1.7e, an mA of 4 (four times) the original value should be selected if the image is repeated (as used for the image in Fig. 1.7c, which was obtained using an optimal exposure).

GEOMETRY OF IMAGE PRODUCTION

The objective of diagnostic imaging is to produce images of optimum quality for diagnosis and to aid in the management/treatment of the patient. The ideal set up is to have the body part (object) being imaged parallel to and in contact with the image detector. The X-ray beam should be at right angles to the detector and not angled across it, as this produces a distorted image. However, there are situations where the patient or X-ray beam is angled to deliberately distort/elongate the image, such as a 30-degree angled elongated scaphoid projection (see Fig. 2.67b).

All radiographic images produced using an X-ray source (focus) and detector will be projected larger than the object being imaged. However, this is not always apparent from the image on the monitor as the image is optimised for image viewing by the computing system and may appear life size. There are some important aspects determined by the geometry of the imaging system which are relevant when producing the image:

- magnification;
- unsharpness;
- resolution/definition.

All of these factors affect the image when positioning the patient and selecting the equipment for X-ray examination. Table 1.2 states terms related to geometry.

One key skill of the radiographer is to produce images with minimal magnification and unsharpness. Any unsharpness produced by the technique is magnified by the object-to-receptor distance (ORD). Magnification is reduced by close contact between the patient's body part and the image receptor. In practice, a standardised focus-to-receptor distance (FRD) should be used. An FRD of 110 cm for table work and 180 cm for erect chest images is used (Fig. 1.8). FRD distances must be standardised within departments to standardise magnification.

All images produced in radiography have a level of unsharpness, which should not be visible to the radiographer. This is approximately 0.3 mm and is affected by the positioning of the patient, detector and X-ray tube. To minimise geometric unsharpness:

- A fine focus should be used where possible.
- The object (part being X-rayed) should be as close to the detector as possible (ideally in contact).
- The FRD should be as long as practicable as this minimises the penumbra, hence unsharpness. NB: Images with visible unsharpness are not diagnostic and need to be repeated.

The area of the patient irradiated can be controlled by collimation of the X-ray beam. The maximum field size at 100 cm FRD is 43 cm². However, it is critical that the beam of radiation is limited only to the area of interest. This can improve image quality and reduce the radiation dose to the patient, and therefore staff, by minimising the amount of scattered radiation produced.

In direct digital radiography the detector size must be large enough for all radiographic examinations. Most equipment has an active area of at least 43 × 43 cm. Wi-Fi detectors may be provided in smaller sizes, but the resolution is similar to a fixed detector.

Table 1.2 Terms related to geometry.

Distance	Abbreviation
Focus-to-receptor distance	FRD
Focus-to-object distance	FOD
Object-to-receptor distance	ORD

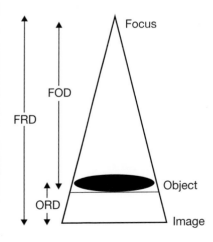

Fig. 1.8 Names of the distances used in radiographic image production.

PATIENT JOURNEY AND EXAMINATION TIMELINE

Successful radiography is dependent on many factors but uppermost is the patient's experience during their short journey and encounter with the diagnostic imaging department. The radiographer has a duty of care to the patient and must treat them with respect and ensure their dignity is maintained. It is essential that the radiographer establishes a rapport with the patient and any carers. The radiographer must introduce themselves to the patient/carer and inform them of their role in the examination. They must make sure the request form is for the patient being examined and that the clinical details and history are accurate. The radiographer must request consent from the patient and the patient must give consent for the examination before the radiographer starts examination.

Figure 1.9 outlines the patient journey and examination timeline. The figure demonstrates a systematic way of undertaking an X-ray examination and ensures that the patient journey is patient-focused and that mistakes are eliminated. The key aspects are:

- effective communication with patients and carers;
- the ability to follow a logical framework to be able to perform the X-ray examination proficiently and effectively;
- efficient use of technology to produce diagnostic images at the first attempt;
- evaluation of the radiographic image using the 10-point plan.

Stages of an X-ray Procedure

There are three stages to undertaking an X-ray examination: preparation, the X-ray examination itself and follow-up from the procedure undertaken. Each of these stages can be further subdivided as shown here and in Fig. 1.9.

Preparation for the Procedure

- checks for the referral and justification for the request;
- the equipment and environment;
- preparation of the patient, staff and carers, including consent for the examination and identity checks.

Undertaking the Procedure

- patient care and management;
- radiographic procedure;
- radiation protection.

Post X-ray Procedure

- patient and staff aftercare;
- image quality;
- imaging informatics.

Although there are several 'main headings' to the algorithm it is essential to emphasise that the primary focus is the patient and their interaction within the process.

Communication

Communication can take place in several ways: verbal, non-verbal and visual. Communication should be clear from the first contact with patients, carers and staff. A clear and confident communication style is needed with lack of ambiguity or jargon, especially when communicating with the patient.

Effective communication encompasses a myriad of interactions which include being open and friendly to the patient, telling them who you are, what you are intending to do, gaining consent and also inviting and answering any questions they may have about the examination. Figure 1.10 gives guidelines to demonstrate effective communication from the radiographer to the patient.

The radiographer should verify that the patient has understood the information and instructions provided. They must ensure that the patient consents to having the X-ray examination performed. It is important that radiographers must communicate when patients are unresponsive and/or unconscious. When it is not possible to clearly seek and obtain consent from the patient directly, due to an underlying medical condition, mental state or lack of competence, such consent is to be sought and obtained by a legal representative on the patient's behalf. Take your time to speak to those looking after the patient, such as a parent, carer or healthcare professional. They will be able to assist you with identification checks and give you an insight into the patient's likes and dislikes, which will give you an idea as to how to carry out the examination.

Preparation

Checks for the referral

Review:
- Imaging request to make sure it is authorised and justified
- Previous studies and consider images/reports
- Department protocols and decide if any modifications to the technique are required

Identify
- Infection risk
- Wear appropriate PPE for COVID 19 patients
- Radiation protection requirements
- Any patient specific needs
- Department protocols and decide if any modifications to the technique are required

Equipment and environment

- Ensure imaging equipment is subject to regular QC testing
- Room clean and tidy
- Equipment set up in preparation for the study to be undertaken
- Contrast Agent prepared, checked and recorded as required
- Establish the imaging examination is within the protocol/regulations for procedures
- Consider any contraindications or confounding factors

Preparation of the patient, staff and carer

- Communicate effectively with patient staff and carers
- Explain what you are there to do and the procedure
- Hello my name is …
- Check pregnancy status if person of child bearing capacity
- Obtain consent for the examination by giving a clear explanation to include any benefits/risk
- Explain any specific preparations for the X-ray procedure e.g. identify artefacts which may need to be removed

Have you paused and checked?

Procedure

Patient care and management

- Visibly wash/clean your hands
- Communicate effectively and give clear instructions
- Be open and approachable
- Explain what you are doing
- Explain why you are doing it
- Invite any questions and reply within the scope of your practice

Radiographic Procedure

- Ensure the patient is identified correctly
- Ensure the correct procedure is about to be carried out
- Decide on the protocol and any modifications required
- Work safely and efficiently
- Consider distract or immobilisation techniques
- Get a diagnostic image at first attempt

Radiation Protection

- Adhere to local rules
- Confirm the appropriate protocol
- Only essential staff present
- Utilise appropriate PPE e.g. lead rubber aprons
- Optimise the exposure
- **Apply the principles of radiation protection**
- Time

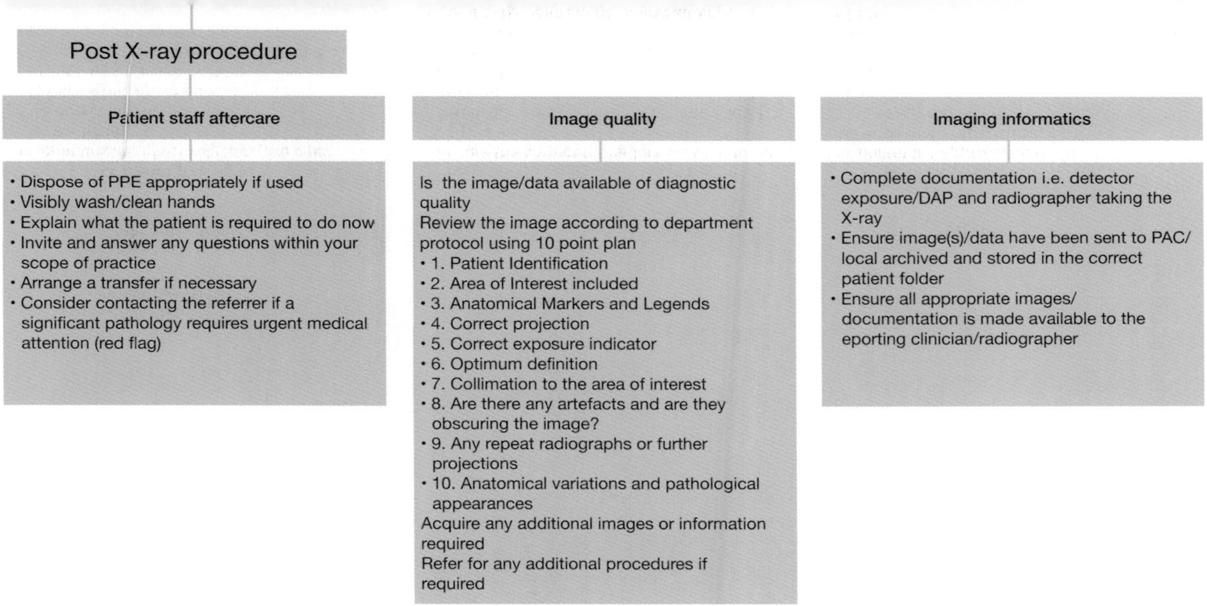

Post X-ray procedure

Patient staff aftercare

- Dispose of PPE appropriately if used
- Visibly wash/clean hands
- Explain what the patient is required to do now
- Invite and answer any questions within your scope of practice
- Arrange a transfer if necessary
- Consider contacting the referrer if a significant pathology requires urgent medical attention (red flag)

Image quality

Is the image/data available of diagnostic quality

Review the image according to department protocol using 10 point plan
- 1. Patient Identification
- 2. Area of Interest included
- 3. Anatomical Markers and Legends
- 4. Correct projection
- 5. Correct exposure indicator
- 6. Optimum definition
- 7. Collimation to the area of interest
- 8. Are there any artefacts and are they obscuring the image?
- 9. Any repeat radiographs or further projections
- 10. Anatomical variations and pathological appearances

Acquire any additional images or information required

Refer for any additional procedures if required

Imaging informatics

- Complete documentation i.e. detector exposure/DAP and radiographer taking the X-ray
- Ensure image(s)/data have been sent to PAC/ local archived and stored in the correct patient folder
- Ensure all appropriate images/ documentation is made available to the eporting clinician/radiographer

Fig. 1.9 Patient journey and examination timeline. DAP, dose-area product.

25

Patient communication

Greet the patient and introduce yourself to them

Hello my name is Ken

I am a radiographer

Please may I ask your name and date of birth

How would you like to be addressed?

Explain why you are there, your role in the examination and provide clear instructions/information about what needs to be done

I am here to take your X-ray/perform your examination

It will not hurt and will not take long (give an estimate of the time)

This is what I would like you to do ....

Is that OK with you?

Gain consent and engage in a benefit/risk dialogue

This X-ray examination will help us find out what's wrong with you (make a diagnosis) so we can provide you with the correct care and treatment

The benefits of the procedure are greater than the small risk associated with the use of X-rays

My role is to perform the examination with the minimum radiation dose and minimise any risk

Please can I take your X-ray/perform your examination?

Offer relevant information, wish the patient well and thank them

This X-ray examination is finished and I will now send the images/data for reporting (or I will report them)

The results will take .... (give a timeframe)

Thank you for your cooperation/help

Take care/keep well

Fig. 1.10 Guidelines for effective communication from the radiographer to the patient.

GENERAL CONSIDERATIONS FOR DIGITAL RADIOGRAPHIC EXAMINATIONS

Patient Considerations

- Always introduce yourself to the patient and state your profession.
- Explain the procedure and the patient's role.
- Rehearse any breathing manoeuvres (or similar) if the patient has a limited ability to cooperate.
- Check if the patient has complied with any preparation instructions (e.g. have they removed relevant clothing or jewellery?).
- Ask if the patient has any questions or concerns.
- After the examination inform the patient what they should do next and check they understand the advice given.

Procedural Considerations

- Always prepare the X-ray room for the procedure prior to the patient entering the room.
- Follow departmental protocols for the examination, e.g. the FRD, which is normally 110 cm unless otherwise stated.
- Always collimate to the area of interest as excessive field sizes reduce image quality and increase patient dose.
- It is best practice to apply anatomical side markers at the time of the examination and not to use electronic markers when post-processing the image.

Imaging Informatics

In respect to imaging informatics, it is important that the acquired images are viewed carefully using optimised conditions, i.e. that the department/manufacturer recommendations regarding any specific algorithms associated with a body part have been followed and any further post-processing has been carefully considered before the images are sent to the PACS.

The exposure must be optimised and recorded to evaluate the patient's exposure and ensure there is minimal/no noise on the image. Exposure details, dose reading and number of images taken is recorded on the RIS (including rejected images). Exposure and dose readings may also be recorded on the image itself.

PATIENT IDENTITY AND CONSENT

Introduction

It is essential that the radiographer establishes a rapport with the patient and carers. The radiographer must first introduce themselves and inform the patient/carer what to expect during the examination. Then they must make sure the request form is for the patient being examined and the clinical details and history are accurate. The patient/carer's consent must be requested before the examination starts.

Request Form

The radiographer checks the request form to ensure the examination is justified according to:

- the Ionising Radiation (Medical Exposure) Regulations (IR(ME)R) 2017 (amended in 2018):
- department protocols, making sure all the required details are on the form, i.e. patient demographics, examination requested, authorised signature for the examination and an explanation of the examination requested;
- the clinical details provided by the referring clinician.

Patient Identity and Consent

- Patient identity is established using departmental protocol, which normally requires you to ask the patient to state their full name, address and date of birth. These are then cross-referenced with the request form. The examination must not proceed unless the radiographer is sure of the identity of the patient.
- The procedure is explained to the patient in easy to understand terms avoiding medical jargon.

The patient is asked:

- if they have undertaken any required preparation for the examination;
- if they understand the nature of the examination and if they have any questions prior to proceeding;
- for verbal permission to proceed with the examination;

- for written consent if an examination incurs a higher risk, e.g. angiography.

To be able to give consent (whether an adult or child) the patient should meet the following criteria:

- they should understand the benefits and risk of the examination;
- they should understand the nature of the examination and why it is being performed;
- they should understand the consequences of not having the examination;
- they should be able to make and communicate an informed decision.

If these conditions are not fulfilled then other individuals may be able to give consent, e.g. parents, or in an emergency situation the examination may proceed if it is considered in the best interest of the patient (refer to the hospital's policy).

JUSTIFICATION FOR THE EXAMINATION

Upon receipt of a referral for an X-ray examination, the radiographer needs to carefully consider if the requested examination is appropriate to undertake. In other words – is the examination justified?

The radiographer should consider several questions when assessing any request for imaging.

- **Will the examination change the clinical management of the patient?**
  Although this can be a contentious area, the radiographer should consider whether the requested examination will be of benefit to the patient and whether the findings will affect the patient's treatment or management.

- **Does the completed request comply with local protocol?**
  For example, is the request card completed in a legible manner? Are the patient demographics correct? Is the requested examination in line with departmental protocol? Is the referrer identified and working within their referral protocol?

- **Are the details of previous operations or other relevant recent imaging included?**
  This may have a bearing on the projections taken or the validity of the requested examination.

- **What are the benefits and risks of the examination?**
  The benefits of having an X-ray are associated with managing the treatment and/or diagnosis of the patient. These may include the following.
    - saving the person's life by providing the correct diagnosis, which may not be possible without the use of X-rays, e.g. chest X-ray to demonstrate extent of pathology;
    - giving the patient the correct treatment at the correct time as a result of the correct diagnosis;
    - eliminating disease/disorders which affect the management of the patient, e.g. determining if a patient has a fracture and how best to manage it.

The patient should be made aware that the benefits of imaging are greater than the negligible risks associated with the radiation dose delivered. For example, a chest X-ray typically delivers 0.02 mSv, which is similar to about 3 days of background radiation.

The aim of the benefit/risk dialogue is to ensure that patients are appropriately informed and involved. In effect, a dialogue entails that communication occurs in both directions so it is equally important that the radiographer takes the time to stop and listen to the patient. This is essential in further establishing a good rapport with the patient as it provides an opportunity to be heard, have questions answered and/or concerns addressed.

Even low X-ray doses can cause changes to cell DNA, leading to increased probability of cancer occurring in the years following the exposure. Although in many cases the probability of this occurring is low (Table 1.3), the risk should always be balanced against the benefits of the patient undergoing the examination. This is often acutely emphasised when seriously ill patients undergo frequent X-ray examinations and the need to consider each request carefully is very important. Consultation with radiological colleagues may be required if there is any doubt over the legitimacy of any request.

Table 1.3 Radiation risk for X-ray examinations to an average adult.

Examination	Typical effective dose (mSv)	Risk*
Hand/Foot	0.01	1 in a few million
Chest	0.02	1 in 1 000 000
Mammography	0.06	1 in 300 000
Abdomen	0.7	1 in 30 000
Lumbar spine	1.3	1 in 15 000
CT head	2	1 in 10 000
Barium enema	7.2	1 in 2800
CT body	9	1 in 2200

*Additional lifetime risk of fatal cancer.
CT, computed tomography.

- **Does the request comply with government legislation?**
Legislation varies between countries; however, the request should comply with national legislation where applicable. In the UK, the underlying legislation is known as the Ionising Radiation (Medical Exposure) Regulations (IR(ME)R) 2017.

  This legislation is intended to protect patients by keeping doses as low as reasonably practicable. The regulations set out responsibilities for those who refer patients for an examination (referrers), those who justify the exposure to take place (practitioners) and those who undertake the exposure (operators). Radiographers frequently act as practitioners and as such must be aware of the legislation along with the benefits and risks of the examination to be able to justify it. The referrer has a legal responsibility to provide sufficient information on the request to enable the practitioner to determine if the examination is justified.

- **Is there an alternative imaging modality?**
The use of an alternative imaging modality, which may provide more relevant information than X-ray or give the required information at a lower radiation dose, should be considered. The information may be provided without a radiation dose at all. The use of non-ionising imaging modalities, such as ultrasound and magnetic resonance (MRI), should be considered where appropriate.

RADIATION PROTECTION

The radiographer has a duty of care to ensure that the exposure delivered to the patient conforms to the departmental optimisation's policy. This ensures that the principle of keeping doses as low as reasonably practicable has been applied. The radiographer also is responsible for the protection of staff and others involved in the use of ionising radiation as well as themselves.

Departments may have the Society of Radiographers pause and check guidelines displayed in X-ray rooms to help with completing the examination safely (see Have you paused and checked? IR(ME)R; https://www.sor.org/learning-advice/professional-body-guidance-and-publications/documents-and-publications/policy-guidance-document-library/have-you-paused-and-checked-ir(me)r).

The following is a list of general principles that can be followed to minimise dose to patients and staff at various stages of the radiological examination.

Patient

- Explain the procedure to the patient and the need to keep still.
- Make the patient comfortable.

Other Staff and Carers

- Only required staff and carers should be in the X-ray room.
- If a carer is supporting the patient, they should be monitored with a radiation monitoring device, and personal protective equipment (PPE) used.

The Radiographer's Role

- Justify the request.
- Optimise the exposure.
- X-ray the correct patient: check three forms of identification (name, address and date of birth).
- X-ray the correct body part: check against body part on the request and the patient history.

- Collimate to the area of interest.
- Use a careful technique (no repeated examinations).
- Use optimum exposure factors (DRLs are a legal requirement of practice).
- Optimum beam energy (kV) should be used for the examination and imaging system.
- Stand behind the radiation barrier when the exposure is made.
- Do not point the X-ray tube in the direction of the radiation barrier or doors (which must be closed).

Additional Considerations

- Prepare the room and set a preliminary exposure before inviting the patient into the X-ray room.
- Always explain what you are trying to achieve and what is expected of the patient.
- Equipment must have regular QA checks to ensure it is working at the optimum level.
- If a patient is worried about the radiation dose they might receive you can use the following statements to put the risk into context.
    - 'You have more chance of drowning in the bath in the next year than you have of getting cancer from a chest/extremity X-ray.'
    - 'An abdomen X-ray carries about the same risk of death as playing a game of football.'
    - 'A computed tomography (CT) head examination carries approximately the same risk of death that the average UK road user faces per year.'

Optimisation of the Exposure

The IR(ME)R 2017 regulations state that 'The practitioner and the operator, to the extent of their respective involvement in a medical exposure, shall ensure that radiation doses arising from the exposure are kept as low as reasonably practicable consistent with the intended purpose.' The regulations also state that that the operator shall select equipment and methods to ensure that for each medical exposure the dose of ionising radiation to the individual undergoing the exposure is as low as reasonably practicable (Table 1.4) and consistent with the intended diagnostic or therapeutic purpose. In doing so, the operator should pay special attention to:

- careful/precise technique to minimise repeat examinations;
- quality assurance of equipment;
- optimisation of exposure factors to provide a diagnostic image within the DRLs set for each procedure;
- agreed exposure in anatomically programmed equipment/exposure charts;
- clinical audit of procedures and exposures.

It is important therefore that special attention is paid to these relevant issues to ensure that patient doses are kept to a minimum.

Table 1.4 Radiation dose quantities.

Dose quantities	Unit	Definition
Absorbed dose	Gy	Energy absorbed in a known mass of tissue
Organ dose	mGy	Average dose to specific tissue
Effective dose	mSv	Overall dose weighted for sensitivity of different organs; indicates risk
Entrance surface dose	mGy	Dose measured at beam entrance surface; used to monitor doses and set DRLs for radiographs
Dose-area product	Gy per cm^2	Product of dose (in air) and beam area; used to monitor doses and set DRLs for examinations

MEDICAL EXPOSURE AND DIAGNOSTIC REFERENCE LEVELS (DRLs)

Employers have a duty under IR(ME)R 2017 to establish DRLs for radiodiagnostic examinations. European reference levels should be considered when setting DRLs. For the UK such levels have been based on a series of national patient dose surveys conducted over the years with the latest report being published in 2022 (https://www.gov.uk/government/publications/diagnostic-radiology-national-diagnostic-reference-levels-ndrls/ndrl). The national DRLs should be considered by employers when setting their local DRLs as required by the IR(ME)R 2017 and the IR(ME)R (Northern Ireland) 2018.

The recommended DRLs for the procedures published are based on rounded third-quartile values of the mean patient doses observed for common X-ray examinations in a nationally representative sample of X-ray rooms.

The doses are expressed as either entrance skin dose (ESD; mGy) or dose-area product (DAP; Gy·cm²) or both. The focus is mainly on the most frequent or relatively higher-dose examinations. Table 1.5 summarises Table 28 of the report in respect of plain radiographic examinations. The report also includes recommended national DRLs for fluoroscopic and interventional procedures.

The DRLs quoted should be used as a reference for comparison with local DRLs. These should be regularly reviewed in light of national guidance or changes in technique and procedures. Additionally, there is a requirement for the employer to undertake appropriate reviews whenever diagnostic levels are consistently exceeded and ensure that corrective action is taken where appropriate. This means that there should be a regular review of patient doses. The operator, i.e. the radiographer, has a legal requirement to optimise the radiation dose and although individual exposures may vary around the DRL, the average for standard patients should comply with the established level.

This edition of *Clark's Pocket Handbook for Radiographers* quotes DRLs for the majority of adult individual radiographs described using the current recommended UK national DRLs (see Table 1.5 and high-lighted with a red box in Section 2) and for those not included DRLs are added (highlighted with a grey box in Section 2) calculated on a regional basis by means of electronic X-ray examination records courtesy of Integrated Radiological Services (IRS) Ltd, Liverpool.

Paediatric DRLs are addressed in the paediatric chapter of *Clark's Positioning in Radiography*, 13th Edition (Whitley et al. 2016). These DRLs are given as a guide and readers are referred to local protocols and procedures, where relevant local DRLs should be in place. Dose monitoring on a national level enables the establishment of DRLs as well as allowing calculation of the dose burden to the population as a whole.

Table 1.5 Recommended national reference doses for individual radiographs on adult patients in the UK, 2022.

Radiograph	ESD per radiograph (mGy)	DAP per radiograph (Gy cm²)
Abdomen AP	4	2.5
Chest AP	0.2	0.15
Chest LAT	0.5	
Chest PA	0.15	0.1
Cervical spine AP		0.15
Cervical spine LAT		0.15
Knee AP	0.3	
Knee LAT	0.3	
Lumbar spine AP	5.7	1.5
Lumbar spine LAT	10	2.5
Pelvis AP	4	2.2
Shoulder AP	0.5	
Skull AP/PA	1.8	
Skull LAT	1.1	
Thoracic spine AP	3.5	1.0
Thoracic spine LAT	7	1.5

NB: All national DRLs listed were adopted in 2016.
AP, antero-posterior; DAP, dose-area product; ESD, entrance skin dose; LAT, lateral; PA, postero-anterior.

STANDARD OPERATING PROCEDURE FOR PATIENTS OF REPRODUCTIVE POTENTIAL

Avoiding Exposure in Pregnancy

Your imaging department should have standard operating procedures setting out the duties and responsibilities for practitioners and operators under the IR(ME)R 2017 regulations for imaging involving the use of ionising radiation on individuals of childbearing potential. Any irradiation of a fetus should be avoided whenever possible and alternative imaging techniques or diagnostic procedures should be considered before a decision is taken to expose an individual of childbearing potential to ionising radiation. Where pregnancy is not necessarily suspected by the patient, checks must be made to ensure that there is no possibility of pregnancy before the operator proceeds with the examination, particularly if the abdomen or pelvic area is to be irradiated.

All individuals of childbearing potential between the ages of 12–55 years must be consulted about the possibility of pregnancy prior to undergoing imaging investigations using ionising radiation. It may be necessary to extend this age range if there is a possibility of pregnancy at younger or older ages. IR(ME)R 2017 includes the requirement to make enquiries of individuals of childbearing potential. This should accurately reflect the diversity of the gender spectrum in the population. If in any doubt ask the patient if there is a possibility they could be pregnant.

Pregnancy Enquiry Procedure

The patient should be asked the date of their last menstrual period. If the possibility of pregnancy exists, order a pregnancy test (e.g. if the patient is to receive substantial pelvic irradiation) and obtain results before the pelvis is irradiated. The practitioner (in consultation with the referrer) should make a determination whether or not to do the X-ray examination based on clinical need. This process has replaced the '28-day rule' and '10-day rule' in most departments; however, an explanation of these rules may be useful, as follows.

For the 28-day rule the examination may proceed if the patient's menstrual period is not overdue or within 28 days of their last period.

For high-dose examinations, for example CT scans on the abdomen, the 10-day rule is applied. It is unlikely that a patient of childbearing potential will become pregnant in the first 10 days of their menstrual cycle. There should be a clearly defined protocol stating which examinations are classed as 'high dose' where the 10-day rule is used.

A flow chart for the pregnancy enquiry procedure is shown in Fig. 1.11.

Evaluating and Minimising the Radiation Risks in Pregnancy

If the examination does proceed, the relatively small radiation risk to the patient and fetus will be outweighed by the benefit of the diagnosis and subsequent treatment of potentially life-threatening or serious conditions. These could present a much greater risk to both parties if left undiagnosed.

To minimise the risks when examining pregnant patients, the radiographer should adopt the following strategies:

- highest imaging speed system available, e.g. 800-speed or equivalent settings for computed radiography/direct digital radiography;
- limiting collimation to area of interest;
- use of the minimum number of exposures to establish a diagnosis;
- use of the radiographic or CT projections that give the lowest doses.

The use of patient gonadal shielding during X-ray-based diagnostic imaging should be discontinued as routine practice.

All accidental or unintended exposures to the fetus must be investigated by the Radiation Protection Advisor, usually assisted by an MPE. Inadvertent fetal exposures also need to be reported to the Care Quality Commission (CQC) to determine what lessons can be learned to prevent the incident happening again.

What gender were you assigned at birth and do you have the potential to become pregnant?

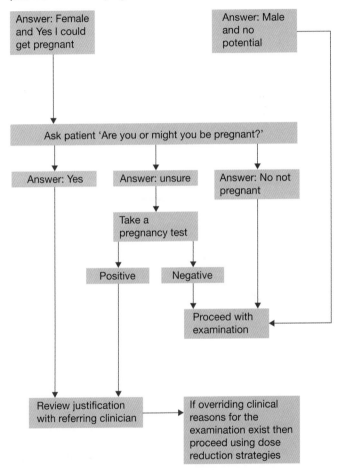

Fig. 1.11 Flow chart for inclusive pregnancy status based on the Society of Radiographers 'Inclusive Pregnancy Guidelines for Ionising Radiation: Diagnostic and Therapeutic Exposures'; SoR 2023.

In the event of an accidental exposure the patient should be counselled and a culture of duty of candour applied (regulation 20) (Care Quality Commission Guidance for Providers; https://www.cqc.org.uk/guidance). According to the International Commission on Radiological Protection (ICRP) pregnancy and medical radiation guidelines (ICRP CRP, 2000. Pregnancy and Medical Radiation. ICRP Publication 84. Ann. ICRP 30 (1)), termination of pregnancy following fetal doses of less than 100 mGy is not justified based upon radiation risk. At fetal doses between 100 and 500 mGy, the decision should be based upon the individual circumstances.

EVALUATING IMAGES: 'THE 10-POINT PLAN'

It is imperative that radiographic images are properly evaluated to ensure that they are fit for purpose, i.e. they must answer the diagnostic question posed by the clinician making the request. To do this effectively the person undertaking the evaluation must be aware of the radiographic appearances of potential pathologies and injuries. They need to understand the relevant anatomy that is demonstrated by a particular projection and the appearances of poor positioning of the patient and equipment. Radiographers should use a standardised process for image review to provide diagnostic-quality images ready for image interpretation.

Points to Consider When Evaluating the Suitability of Radiographic Images

1 **Patient identification**
   Do the details on the image match those on the request card and those of the patient who was examined? Such details will include patient name and demographics, accession number, date and time of examination and the name of the hospital.

2 **Area of interest**
   Does the radiograph include all the relevant areas of anatomy? The anatomy that needs to be demonstrated may vary depending on the clinical indications for the examination.

3 **Markers and legends**
   Check that the correct anatomical side markers are clearly visible in the radiation field. Ensure the marker that has been used matches the body part on the radiographic image and that this in turn matches the initial request from the clinician. Ensure the correct legends have been included if not stated in the examination protocol, such as prone or supine. It is poor practice not to include a marker within the radiation field when making an exposure.

4 **Correct projections**

Does the acquired image follow standard radiographic technique as outlined throughout the book, with the patient being correctly positioned together with the appropriate tube angulation? It is important to consider the pathology/condition in question and the clinical presentation of the patient. If debating whether a projection is acceptable always consider if the diagnostic question has been answered.

5 **Has the correct exposure been given?**

Evaluation of the suitability of the exposure factors used for a radiograph will depend on the equipment and medium used to acquire and capture the image.

Conventional film-/Screen-based imaging

■ *Image density*: the degree of image blackening should allow relevant anatomy to be sufficiently demonstrated, thus allowing diagnosis.

■ *Image contrast*: the range of useful densities produced on the radiographic image should correspond to the structures within the area of interest. Each anatomical area should be of sufficient contrast to allow relevant anatomical structures to be clearly visualised.

Digital image acquisition systems

■ Given the wide exposure latitude of digital systems the primary task when evaluating the image is to assess for over- or underexposure. The imaging equipment will usually give an indication of the exposure used. This may be a numerical exposure indicator. The reading is compared with a range of exposure limits provided by the manufacturer to see if it is above or below recommended values. An alternative method may be a traffic light system to indicate if the exposure is in the required range or if it varies from normal.

■ Unfortunately, these methods are not standardised by the different manufacturers.

Underexposure: images that are underexposed will show unacceptable levels of 'noise' or 'mottle' even though the computer screen brightness (image density) will be acceptable (Fig. 1.12a).

Optimum exposure: images with the correct exposure will have little/no noise and no burnout (excessive blackening) from pixel overload.

The range of densities and contrast will allow the anatomical structures to be clearly demonstrated (definition) There should be no visible unsharpness and a high signal-to-noise ratio (Fig. 1.12b).

Overexposure: image quality will actually improve as exposure increases due to lower levels of noise. However, once a certain point is reached, further increases in exposure will result in reduced contrast. Eventually a point is reached when the image contrast becomes unacceptable (Fig. 1.12c).

NB: There is considerable scope for exposing patients to unnecessarily high doses of radiation using digital imaging technologies. When evaluating images, it is important to always use the lowest dose that gives an acceptable level of image noise. The EI must be in the appropriate range and must be within the national and local DRLs.

(a)   (b)   (c)

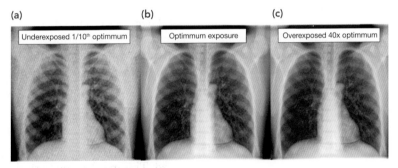

Underexposed 1/10ᵗʰ optimmum   Optimmum exposure   Overexposed 40x optimmum

Fig. 1.12 (a) Underexposed image; (b) optimum image; (c) overexposed image.

6 **Optimum definition**
  Is the image sharp? Look at bone cortices and trabeculae to ensure movement or other factors have not caused an unacceptable degree of image unsharpness.
7 **Collimation to the area of interest**
  Has any of the area of interest been overlooked due to over-collimation? Check relevant soft tissues have been included. Also, look for signs of collimation to evaluate the success of the collimation strategy used. This can then be used for future reference

when performing similar examinations. Collimation outside the area of interest will increase both the radiation dose and image noise (due to increased scattered photons).

8 **Artefacts**

Are there any artefacts on the image and are they obscuring the image? These may be from the patient, their clothing, the equipment or the imaging process. Only repeat if the artefact is interfering with diagnosis.

9 **Need for repeat radiographs or further projections**

A judgement is made from evaluations 1–8. If one or more factors have reduced the diagnostic quality to a point where a diagnosis cannot be made, the image should be repeated. Would any additional projections enhance the diagnostic potential of the examination, such as radial head projections for an elbow radiograph? If a repeat is required it may be appropriate to image only the area where there was uncertainty in the initial image. Would suggesting a referral of the patient for any additional procedures (e.g. ultrasound/CT) enhance the patient outcomes?

10 **Anatomical variations and pathological appearances**

Note anything unusual such as normal variants or pathology that may influence your future actions (see point 9) or aid diagnosis. For example, if an old injury is seen it may be worth questioning the patient about their medical history. This could then be recorded to aid diagnosis.

GUIDELINES FOR THE ASSESSMENT OF TRAUMA IMAGES

Background

Radiographers are well placed to offer opinions on trauma plain radiographic images and can assist the referring clinician with identification of fractures, dislocations and associated 'signs', such as fluid levels. In the UK the practice of 'red-dotting' is well established and involves the radiographer placing a red dot or similar marker on the image to indicate the presence of an abnormality.

Developments in the Role of the Radiographer

In the UK, the basic system of placing a red dot has developed into a three-tier system of radiographer opinion, as follows.

1 **Red dot**: a basic system of flagging a possible abnormality, such as a fracture.
2 **Comment system**: the radiographer attaches a simple comment to the image to explain their concern.
3 **Clinical report**: trained radiographers produce a detailed report, usually sometime after the examination, that is sent to the referring clinician.

Most radiographers, especially newly qualified practitioners, will be working to develop their skills on the red-dot and commenting systems.

Suggestions for Successful Image Evaluation

1 **Gain an oral clinical history:** obtaining a clinical history from the patient can be especially helpful for the radiographer to produce the correct projections required to demonstrate the injury or pathology, as well as a greater understanding of the area to check for injury. Modern PACS also allow the radiographer to convey any relevant clinical history to the person providing the final radiological report.

2 **Produce high-quality radiographs:** poor images are especially difficult to interpret and the ability to exclude fractures with confidence is diminished.

3 **Use a logical system for checking:** many different approaches to evaluating radiographs are suggested in the radiology literature, such as looking at alignment, then bones, followed by cartilage, etc.

  Many useful lines and measurements are used to check for abnormalities, such as McGrigor's three lines for evaluating the facial bones. Whichever system you use, try to apply it consistently and logically, which should reveal many subtle injuries.

4 **Utilise a system of pattern recognition:** carefully trace the cortical outlines of each bone, looking for any steps, breaks or discontinuities. Radiographers are used to seeing a large volume of 'normal' examinations and variants. They are therefore well placed to use this knowledge to identify any changes in the normal pattern of bones and joints. After checking the cortical margins, carefully assess the cancellous components of the bones, looking for discontinuities in the trabecular pattern which may indicate a fracture.

5 **Pay attention to 'hot-spots':** these are where frequent bony injuries occur, such as the neck of the fifth metacarpal, the base of the fifth metatarsal, the dorsal aspect of the distal radius or the supracondylar region of the humerus in children. Frequently, the way the patient presents or reacts to positioning gives strong clues as to the position of the injury.

6 **Be aware of the indirect signs of a fracture:** for example, be able to identify and recognise the significance of an elbow joint effusion or a lipohaemarthrosis (fat/blood interface within the knee or shoulder joint), which can be associated with an underlying fracture. A joint effusion is the presence of increased intra-articular fluid, often seen on radiographs of the elbow and knee by visualising the elevated fat pads adjacent to the joint capsule.

7 **Look for a second fracture:** there is an old saying, 'if you spot one fracture, look for another'. A common mistake is to identify a fracture but miss a second by not checking the entire image. Be aware of principles such as the 'bony ring rule', which states that if a fracture or dislocation is seen within a bony ring (e.g.

pelvis), then a further injury should be sought as there are frequently two fractures.

8 **Add a ball bearing:** when there is a need to assess magnification within the image and calculate the real size of structures, use a scaling ball bearing measuring device. This will assist specialist orthopaedic imaging software to accurately determine suitable prosthesis size in preoperative planning.

THEATRE RADIOGRAPHY

Introduction

Theatre radiography plays a significant role in the delivery of surgical services. The radiographer may be required for emergency procedures or planned surgery in both trauma and non-trauma procedures.

Considerations for the radiographer include the following.

Key Skills for Theatre

Key skills for the radiographer in theatre are:
- how to use the equipment correctly;
- effective communication;
- personal preparation;
- safe practice;
- production of diagnostic images;
- radiation protection of the staff and patients;
- infection control and PPE;
- teamworking.

Effective Use of the Equipment

A mobile X-ray unit or mobile fluoroscopy unit is selected, depending on the requirement of the radiographic procedure. For example, a mobile X-ray unit may be used for plain chest radiography, whereas a mobile fluoroscopy unit may be used for the screening of orthopaedic procedures such as hip pinning.

A mobile fluoroscopy unit should be assembled and tested ahead of the procedure to ensure that it is functioning effectively prior to patient positioning.

Effective Communication

Communication can take place in several ways: verbal, non-verbal and visual. Effective communication must take place between theatre staff and the radiographer, starting with receipt of the request for an examination. This helps the radiographer to be prepared for each examination by understanding the urgency of it, the imaging environment – which will inform the need for appropriate accessories – and the reason for the examination.

The radiographer must maintain a close liaison with all people in the team undertaking the operation, consequently working as part of the multidisciplinary team.

The radiographer must be familiar with the layout and protocols associated with the theatre to which they are assigned, demonstrate a working knowledge of the duties of each person in the operating theatre and ascertain the specific requirements of the surgeon who is operating.

Prior to the operation, communication with the patient should start with a friendly introduction, stating your name and job role and a summary of what the expected outcome will be. If the patient can respond, the radiographer must check that they understand the reason for the examination, confirm their identity and give consent for the examination.

Personal Preparation

Personal preparation is the first concern of the radiographer before entering an aseptic controlled area. The radiographer removes their uniform (and any jewellery) and replaces them with theatre scrubs. If PPE is required for a patient with COVID-19, the hair is covered completely with a disposable hat. Theatre shoes or boots are worn, and a facemask/ventilator is put on. In addition, a radiation-monitoring badge is pinned to theatre garments.

Special attention is made to washing the hands using soap, ensuring that the hands are washed before and after each patient. Skin abrasions should be covered with waterproof dressings.

Image receptor holders, stationary grids and other imaging devices should be cleaned and checked if required.

Contrast media, if required, should also be supplied to the theatre staff.

Time Out

It is now common practice in operating theatres to call a 'time out' with the operating team before the operation starts. The procedure is used to stop any errors being made in the procedure and to discuss any issues or anticipated safety concerns, such as patient allergies or anticipated complications. The points listed below are checked in the presence of the surgeon, operating nurse, anaesthetist and radiographer. It is usual to have the signed consent form from the patient and a wristband on the patient as a reference point.

Preoperative checks include:

- patient identification;
- signed consent for the procedure;
- the operation being undertaken and the relevant anatomical side;
- negative methicillin-resistant *Staphylococcus aureus* (MRSA) and COVID-19 tests;
- pregnancy check if appropriate;
- previous radiographic images on PACS.

PACS Connectivity

In many theatre suites it is customary for the X-ray equipment to be housed within the suite. A PACS/digital imaging and communications in medicine link should be established to facilitate image capture and retrieval of previous examinations. This may be on a separate PACS link in the theatre. Patients need to be entered prior to the procedure commencing to allow the images to be acquired and stored in the correct files.

Radiation Protection

Radiation protection is the responsibility of the radiographer operating the X-ray equipment. Therefore, the radiographer should ensure that radiation monitoring badges, lead protective aprons and thyroid shields are worn by all staff when in the controlled area (2 m from the X-ray tube). Furthermore, as soon as the imaging equipment is switched on, a controlled area exists (Ionising Radiations Regulations [IRR] 2017 regulation 17). Therefore, all doors giving access to the controlled area must display radiation warning signs. Personnel not required for the procedure must leave the theatre when an exposure is made.

The key points are as follows.

- Patient identification must be confirmed with either the anaesthetist or an appropriate member of the theatre team prior to commencement of image acquisition, or with the patient if they are awake.

- The radiographer should not be surprised if the surgeon wants to screen while rotating the limb or during a dynamic screwing. Fluoroscopy is a dynamic process and if dynamic images are not required then it would be better to use a digital mobile X-ray unit as the image quality is better. However, this is rarely done due to chances of cross infection.
- Focused collimation to the area of interest when using fluoroscopy will reduce radiation dose and scatter, improving image quality. C-arm units generally have sufficient resolution for theatre imaging requirements.
- The inverse square law must be applied in the theatre environment. Therefore, staff must be standing at the maximum distance from the source of radiation, and outside the path of the radiation field during exposure.
- The radiographer must limit the dose to the patient and staff by use of dose-saving facilities (variable fluoroscopic pulse rates) and by minimising fluoroscopy times. Fluoroscopy should only be undertaken when the surgeon indicates that it is required and has done something to the patient since the previous screen.
- The radiographer must give clear instructions to staff before any exposures are made regarding their role, to reduce the risk of accidental exposure. They may also need to give advice to the clinician undertaking the screening, if appropriate.
- It is a legal requirement to record the screening time and radiation dose for each patient examination. The records should be monitored regularly to ensure the doses are as low as reasonably practicable and conform to local DRLs.

Sterile Procedures/Infection Prevention and Control

Equipment used in operating theatres must be kept clean and stored in the theatre environment. It must be cleaned regularly and prior to and after every case. Not all theatre cases require full sterile protection so the equipment should be protected appropriately and covered to shield the patient from infection and the equipment from damage.

When a sterile procedure is required and in all invasive procedures where the skin is pierced a mobile fluoroscopy unit must be covered appropriately by sterile plastic coverings or drapes. Sterile procedures are an everyday occurrence for the theatre staff so their help and guidance can easily be sought. The radiographer should avoid the contamination of sterile areas. Ideally, equipment should be positioned before any sterile towels are placed in position and care should be exercised not to touch sterile areas when positioning the C-arm component or moving equipment during the operation, unless it is draped.

Personal Protective Equipment (PPE)

PPE must be worn when carrying out mobile examinations when contact may be made with the patient or their surroundings. It must be changed between each patient.

Dependent on the level of risk, PPE can comprise:

- surgical mask to be worn when in close contact with a patient;
- filtering face piece (FFP3) respirator if a procedure involves the generation of aerosols or in cases of possible COVID-19 infection, such as when undertaking cardiopulmonary resuscitation or some surgical procedures;
- plastic apron when in close contact with a patient;
- a gown which must be worn when aerosol-generating procedures are taking place or with patients who potentially have COVID-19;
- gloves, which do not need to be sterile unless carrying out a sterile procedure;
- eye protection if there is a risk of contamination from droplets, such as those released when a patient coughs or sneezes, for example; eye protection can be in the form of protective glasses, goggles or face shield.

PPE should be donned (put on) and doffed (taken off) in a particular way so that maximum protection is received, and the risk of self-contamination is reduced during removal. Local training should be accessed, but the important aspects to remember are that the facemask is the last element to be removed and hands must be washed prior to touching the mask, using the ear loops or ties only. Hands must be washed again after removing and disposing of the mask.

WARD RADIOGRAPHY

Radiography using mobile X-ray equipment should be restricted to the patient whose medical condition is such that it is impossible for them to be moved to the X-ray department without seriously affecting their medical treatment and nursing care. The justification guidelines should be reflective of referral guidelines, which offer up-to-date evidence-based guidance to help the clinician to decide what is the best examination for their patient. These may be local guidelines or one of the nationally agreed guidelines, such as the Royal College of Radiologists' iRefer, the European Society of Radiology's iGuide or the American College of Radiology's Appropriateness Criteria. However, despite having justification guidelines and referral guidelines, it is still important to check that the examination you are going to perform is appropriate.

Key Skills for Mobile/Ward Radiography

- how to use the equipment correctly;
- effective communication;
- radiation protection of staff and patients;
- infection control;
- safe practice, e.g. pregnancy status of staff and patients;
- production of diagnostic images;
- teamworking.

General Considerations

- Any referrals should be checked first to ensure that the examination on the ward/emergency department is necessary.
- Patient identification protocols should be correctly applied.
- For the prevention of infection, the unit selected and image detectors should be cleaned and dried before and after each patient. Appropriate PPE should be worn for radiation protection and infection control.

- The radiographer must enlist the help, cooperation and advice of nursing and medical staff before embarking on an examination.
- A thorough knowledge of the ward is necessary so that any problems or difficulties can be resolved with the minimum of delay.
- Advice regarding the patient's medical condition should be sought first, before moving or disturbing the patient.
- Any disturbance of traction, electrocardiogram (ECG) leads or drains should be undertaken only with the permission of the medical staff.
- Positioning of the image receptor and movement or lifting of seriously ill patients should be undertaken with the cooperation/supervision from nursing staff.
- Patients should be undressed appropriately to remove clothing artefacts.
- Patients should be positioned carefully without rotation and with the sagittal plane in the middle of the image detector.
- The correct mobile equipment and detectors need to be transferred to the ward/emergency department ready to use for the examination.
- The radiographer must be able to assume total control of the situation.

Correct Use of the Equipment

- A mobile X-ray unit is selected depending upon the requirement of the radiographic procedure. The mobile unit may be situated in an area where mobile examinations can be undertaken on a routine basis or may need to be taken to the ward.
- For the prevention of infection, the unit selected and image detectors should be cleaned and dried before and after each patient.
- Patient demographics should be entered on the radiology information system (RIS) and exposure parameters adjusted to those required for the examination.
- Detectors used must be clearly marked to avoid double exposure if more than one patient needs examining on the ward.

Effective Communication

The radiographer needs to communicate effectively to complete the examination without harming the patient's progress or recovery and with minimum disruption to the management of the ward. The radiographer must communicate effectively with the ward staff before, during and after the mobile X-ray.

The key to a stress-free experience is preparation. It is essential that there is a mechanism for ward staff to communicate effectively and give the radiographer as much notice as possible of all mobile imaging requests. This enables the radiographer to use their time effectively and not be kept waiting due to the patient's or ward management.

The radiographer needs to be informed of the:

- reasons for justification for the examination to be a mobile and how it will influence the management of the patient;
- urgency of the request and whether this the correct time for the examination;
- patient's condition and any life support equipment being used;
- infection status, especially with regard to potential COVID-19 infection.

Following the procedure the radiographer must ensure the image(s) are of diagnostic quality. They may give a preliminary assessment/report if it is part of the protocol. The ward staff and referrer must be informed when the image will be available on the PACS. All exposures require clinical evaluation under the IR(ME)R 2017 regulations.

Red Flags

If the X-ray examination of the patient demonstrates a life-threatening or unexpected appearance (e.g. a nasogastric tube in the lung rather than the stomach) the radiographer has a duty of care to the patient and the referrer. The ward and clinician should be informed immediately.

Radiation Protection

This is of paramount importance in the situation where mobile radiography is undertaken.

- The radiographer is responsible for ensuring that there is a controlled area of 2 m during exposure of the patient and that the local rules are adhered to during the examination.
- The radiographer must liaise clearly with the ward staff on their arrival on the ward and issue verbal instructions in a clear and distinct manner to staff and patients to avoid accidental exposure to radiation.
- Anyone assisting in an examination must be protected adequately from scatter radiation by the use of PPE. The use of the inverse square law, with staff standing as far away as possible from the unit and outside the controlled area, should be applied when making an exposure. If a horizontal beam technique is being used the beam should be directed away from staff.

The patient should also receive appropriate radiation protection. Lead protective shields may be used as backstops when using a horizontal beam to limit the radiation field, such as when the absorption nature of room-dividing walls is unknown. Exposure factors used for the examination should be recorded, enabling optimum results to be repeated. Patients tend to be X-rayed frequently when under intensive care.

Control of Infection

The control of infection plays an important role in the management of all patients, especially following surgery and in the nursing of premature babies.

To prevent the spread of infection, local established protocols should be adhered to by staff coming into contact with patients, e.g. hand-washing before and after every patient. Also, detectors and X-ray equipment used for radiographic examination must be cleaned before, between and after each examination. Patients with a known highly contagious infection, and those with a compromised immune system and at high risk of infection, will be isolation-nursed (barrier-nursed; see below). In such circumstances, it is important that local protocols associated with the prevention of spread of infection are followed.

The X-ray equipment used in intensive care units (ICUs), cardiac surgery units and special care baby units should, ideally, be dedicated equipment and kept on site. If shared with other areas in the hospital they should be cleaned with disinfectant solution before being moved into infection-controlled units. Equipment is wheeled over dust-absorbent mats at the entrance of such units.

Radiographers should wear gowns or disposable plastic aprons, face-masks and over-shoes before entering these areas. Image receptors should be cleaned and covered with plastic sheets or clean pillowcases/towels before use. After use, image receptors and all equipment should be cleaned with antiseptic solution. Disposable gloves are worn when touching the patient.

MRSA and *Clostridium difficile* cause hospital-acquired bacterial infections that need to be controlled and not spread to other patients. MRSA is resistant to methicillin and many other antibiotics and is a particular threat to vulnerable patients. It can cause many symptoms, including fever, wound and skin infections, inflammation and pneumonia. Both diseases can be spread readily from an infected patient to others. They are spread mainly from person to person by hand.

When healthcare workers deal with a potentially infected patient, the bacteria may transfer to their hands and can then be passed on to a vulnerable patient. At-risk patients need to be isolation- or barrier-nursed. Controls such as effective hand-washing, wearing of gloves and aprons, and the cleaning of the environment and equipment are necessary to prevent the spread of bacteria.

When undertaking radiography on more than one barrier-nursed patient on a ward or ICU, it is important that disposable aprons are changed between patients as well as ensuring that the hands of the operators are washed between patients to prevent the spread of infection. A number of speciality wards use different-coloured aprons for each patient bay as a prompt to confine the use of aprons to a specific patient.

Isolation/Barrier Nursing

Source isolation nursing is required to reduce the risk of spreading certain infections or antibiotic-resistant germs to other patients and staff. It is also applied to protect patients from infection if they have a weak immune system due to disease, transplant surgery or when taking certain drugs (protective isolation).

- **Source isolation** is carried out by placing the patient in a single room or side room.

- **Barrier nursing** occurs when a patient is kept in a bay and extra precautions are implemented to prevent spread of infection.

There are specific protocols under which two members of staff undertake the X-ray examination to prevent the spread of infection for patients being isolation-/barrier-nursed.

Both radiographers should introduce themselves to the patient, gain consent and explain the procedure to the patient.

Radiographer 1:

- positions the X-ray equipment and makes the exposure;
- cleans the detector and hands it to radiographer 2 who puts the detector in a clean cover, ready to position under the patient,
- takes the detector from the cover after the exposure and cleans it again.

Radiographer 2:

- applies an anatomical marker to the detector;
- positions the patient and detector ready for the exposure;
- hands the detector back to radiographer 1 for processing and checking of the diagnostic quality of the image before leaving the ward;
- makes the patient comfortable and answers any questions.

COVID-19 Patients

In the COVID-19 pandemic chest radiography played a role in detecting changes in the lungs. In the context of COVID-19-positive patients, or those suspected of having the infection, who require imaging, the primary message that all radiographers should aim to convey is one of reassurance. Patients are likely to be fearful, anxious, isolated and sad and therefore they need to be reassured that they are not alone. Therefore, whereas it is understandable that the radiographer may also be anxious or fearful when they need to image a COVID-19-positive or -suspected patient, it is important that the radiographer shows that they truly care and are there to support the patient. Such an approach exhibits a good first impression and paves the way for a positive start for the subsequent radiographer–patient interaction.

The inclusion of a photo of yourself on the outside of your PPE in a transparent cover can add a personal perspective for the patient. Eye contact is hugely important in patient interactions and so the inability of a patient to see our faces and facial expressions is a major loss when full PPE is in use. The photo identifies you and tells the patient who is taking the image. See the earlier section on 'Theatre Radiography' for more information on PPE for COVID-19 patients.

BARIATRIC IMAGING

The worldwide increases in the prevalence of obesity present radiographers with significant challenges when undertaking diagnostic imaging using projectional radiography techniques. These issues can be broadly broken down into four general areas. It is beyond the scope of this text to provide specific advice for each examination but if the radiographer follows some general principles related to each of the four areas, described below, it will assist in optimising image quality and the patient experience. The key to success in this field of imaging is forward planning and communication with the patient, their family and all agencies involved with their care.

Patient Positioning and Transport (Practical Motion)

Transporting the patient to the imaging department and moving them onto the imaging equipment presents a significant risk of musculoskeletal injury to the radiographer. This can be compounded by the fact that many patients struggle to cooperate and achieve the correct position when undertaking an imaging procedure. Following the guidelines below will mitigate this risk.

- Do not exceed personal manual handling limits for lifting, e.g. the limb of a bariatric patient can easily exceed this limit.
- Ensure there are sufficient mechanical lifting aids available in the imaging department.
- Forward plan for examinations and ensure procedures are in place for alerting the department when a bariatric patient requires an examination.
- Ensure there are sufficient staff available, e.g. it may take two individuals to elevate a limb.
- Audit working procedures and learn from incidents, e.g. to ensure future budget planning processes include new equipment if it is required.
- Forward thinking is required to ensure the design of facilities are appropriate for bariatric patients.

- Given the difficulty in locating centring points, which can lead to positioning errors, radiographers should constantly reflect upon the success of the adaptions they make when centring the beam for different body parts, for example displacing the centring point to allow for additional adipose tissue.

Equipment Selection

- Always check the weight limits of equipment, ideally well before the procedure has started.
- Ensure the needs of bariatric patients are accounted for when planning to procure equipment and in the design of facilities, e.g. size of cubicles.
- Reflect on and learn from incidents where equipment was not available.
- Ensure adequate supplies of equipment or supplies designed for bariatric patients are always available, e.g. gowns.

Image Quality

For projectional radiographic techniques the key to success lies in the reduction of the additional scatter produced from excess adipose tissue. This has a significant impact on image quality by reducing radiographic contrast. To mitigate the impact of scatter the following strategies can be adopted.

- Use higher-ratio grids for bariatric patients. For instance, the grid in the Bucky of a table or wall stand will have a higher ratio than loose grids that are placed over the image receptor. Higher-ratio grids are very effective at removing more scatter from the beam compared to lower-ratio grids.
- Consider the use of grids in cases where they would not routinely be used, e.g. knee or shoulder examinations.
- Take additional care when centring the beam. As mentioned previously it may be difficult to palpate bony landmarks when positioning. It may be necessary to allow for the presence of additional tissue compared to a technique used on a non-bariatric patient, e.g. to centre several centimetres anteriorly for a lateral lumbar spine due to the additional soft tissue on the posterior surface of the patient's trunk.

- Always reflect upon the success of centring techniques used for bariatric patients and make adjustments as appropriate for future examinations if sub-optimal images are produced.
- Always evaluate the digital dose indicator to assess if the correct exposure has been achieved. It is easy to position an ionisation chamber incorrectly if bony landmarks cannot be felt when positioning.
- Tissue-displacement techniques are a very effective method of increasing image quality, e.g. moving abdominal fat aprons away from the hips or breast tissue from over the lung bases.
- Use compensation filters and tight collimation fields for lateral hip examinations. For example, the Ferlic filter, if used correctly, has a profound positive impact upon image quality for lateral neck of femur examinations in bariatric patients.

When using the light beam diaphragm to select the collimation field it is easy to inadvertently create a larger than intended radiation field on the image receptor. This could be due to the additional soft tissue and size of the patient, meaning the area of the body upon which the light is projected is *closer* to the light beam diaphragm due to the patient's increased size. If the standard/usual collimation field on the surface of the patient is selected the divergent beam will create a larger field size as it has further to travel (diverge) before it interacts with the image receptor. A well-collimated field plays a role in scatter reduction, particularly in bariatric patients. It may therefore help to collimate to the detector before the patient is positioned.

Communicative Stigma

Radiographers may become embarrassed or reluctant to engage with conversations relating to issues caused by obesity. Patients are generally happy to engage with such conversations as long as the radiographer is open and honest about the situation and employs patient-friendly terminology during communications, e.g. say 'we need to move the *soft tissue* from over your abdomen to get a better X-ray' rather than 'we need to move the *fat* from over your abdomen to get a better X-ray'.

Bariatric patients have the same right to respectful and dignified care as any other patient. This can be challenged if staff become frustrated or annoyed if there is a lack of equipment, poor planning or lack of resources. If a patient were to feel a burden or blamed for their condition, then they may be reluctant to engage with the healthcare system in the future.

Figure 1.13 demonstrates a radiograph of both hips taken on a patient on a trolley using a low-ratio stationary grid. Figure 1.14 was taken with the patient on an X-ray table using a higher-ratio grid. The adipose tissue covering the hips was displaced upwards using a thin cotton triangular bandage. Note the improvement in image contrast over the area of interest.

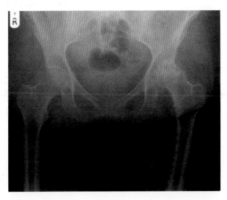

Fig 1.13 Image employing a stationary grid on a trolley.

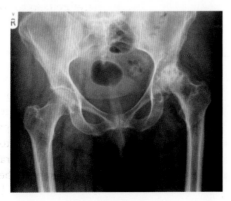

Fig. 1.14 Repeat image taken on an X-ray table using a Bucky and employing upwards displacement of the adipose tissue clear of the area of interest.

SECTION 2
RADIOGRAPHIC PROJECTIONS

ABDOMEN – ANTERO-POSTERIOR SUPINE

Position of Patient and Image Receptor (Fig. 2.1a)

- The patient lies supine on the imaging table with the median sagittal plane at right angles and coincident with the midline of the table.
- The pelvis is adjusted so that the anterior superior iliac spines are equidistant from the table top.
- The detector is placed longitudinally in the Bucky tray (if patient habitus allows) and positioned so that the region below the symphysis pubis is included on the lower margin of the image.
- The centre of the detector will be approximately at the level of a point located 1 cm below the line joining the iliac crests. This will ensure that the region inferior to the symphysis pubis is included on the image.

Direction and Location of the X-ray Beam

- The collimated vertical beam is directed to the centre of the detector to include the lateral margins of the abdomen.
- Using a short exposure time, the exposure is made on arrested respiration. Ideally, respiration should be arrested on full expiration to allow the abdominal contents to lie in their natural position; however, dependent on the patient's height, respiration may need to be arrested on full inspiration to include the whole abdomen.

Essential Image Characteristics (Fig. 2.1b)

- The bowel pattern should be demonstrated with minimal lack of sharpness.

Additional Considerations

- Imaging using a prone position may be employed as a form of compression in the obese patient to reduce patient dose plus the negative effects of scatter upon image quality.
- If available, the use of a virtual grid using direct digital imaging may be employed in situations when the use of a Bucky grid is not possible, i.e. mobile radiography.
- If required, the examination may be undertaken taking two images, with the detector positioned accordingly, to ensure coverage.
- When using an automatic exposure control (AEC) device, the central and right chambers may be selected simultaneously. This is to avoid the risk of underexposure due to the beam passing through regions containing mainly bowel gas.

Expected DRL: DAP 2.5 Gy·cm², ESD 4 mGy*

* DAP, dose-area product; DRL, diagnostic reference level; ESD, entrance skin dose.

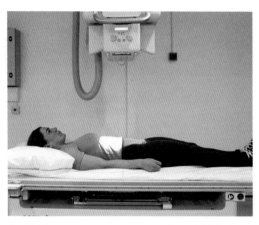

Fig. 2.1a Positioning for an antero-posterior supine projection of the abdomen.

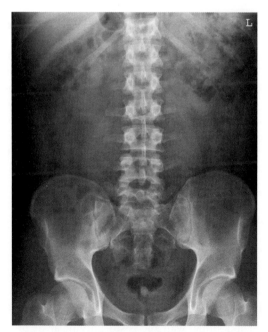

Fig. 2.1b Example of an antero-posterior supine radiograph of the abdomen.

ABDOMEN ANTERO-POSTERIOR – LEFT LATERAL DECUBITUS

This projection is used if the patient cannot be positioned erect for a chest X-ray and is required to confirm the presence of sub-diaphragmatic air. It should only be undertaken as a specific request when other modalities such as ultrasound/computed tomography (CT) cannot be used. It may also be used for confirming a bowel obstruction.

With the patient lying on the left side, free gas will rise to be located between the lateral margin of the liver and the right lateral abdominal wall. To allow time for the gas to collect the patient should remain lying on the left side for a short while (e.g. 10 minutes) before the exposure is made.

Position of Patient and Image Receptor (Fig. 2.2a)

■ The patient lies on their left side, on a trolley or bed, with the elbows and arms flexed so that the hands can rest near the patient's head.
■ The patient is positioned with the posterior aspect of the trunk against a vertical detector/Bucky using a grid engaged with the upper border of the detector, high enough to project above the right lateral abdominal and thoracic walls. Alternatively, a large detector with grid is supported vertically against the patient's back.
■ The patient's position is adjusted to bring the median sagittal plane at right angles to the detector.

Direction and Location of the X-ray Beam

■ The collimated horizontal central beam is directed to the anterior aspect of the patient and centred to the centre of the detector in the midline.

Essential Image Characteristics (Fig. 2.2b)

■ The lateral abdominal wall and costo-phrenic angle of the right lung must be included with the patient resting on their left side for a minimum of 10 minutes prior to exposure.

Expected DRL: DAP 2.5 Gy·cm2, ESD 4 mGy

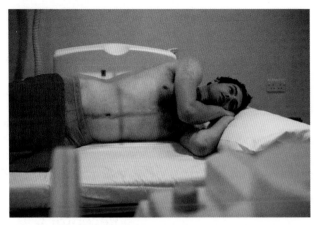

Fig. 2.2a Positioning for an antero-posterior abdomen projection – left lateral decubitus.

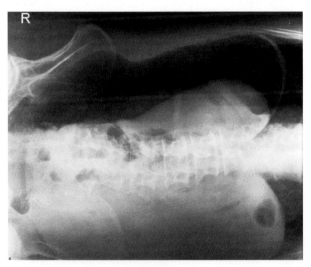

Fig. 2.2b Example of an antero-posterior abdomen radiograph – left lateral decubitus demonstrating free air (perforation).

ACROMIOCLAVICULAR JOINT

Position of Patient and Image Receptor (Fig. 2.3a)

- The patient stands facing the X-ray tube, with the arms relaxed to the side. The shoulder being examined is placed in contact with the detector, and the patient is then rotated approximately 15 degrees towards the side being examined to bring the acromioclavicular joint space at right angles to the detector, with the acromion process central to the field.

Direction and Location of the X-ray Beam

- The collimated horizontal beam is centred to the palpable lateral end of the clavicle at the acromioclavicular joint.
- To avoid superimposition of the joint on the spine of the scapula, the central ray can be angled 15–25 degrees cranially before centring to the joint.

Essential Image Characteristics (Fig. 2.3b)

- The image should demonstrate the acromioclavicular joint and the clavicle aligned with the acromion process of the scapula.
- The image should include soft tissue margins around the joint.

Additional Considerations

- An antero-posterior projection of the joint in question is all that is normally required. However, dependent on the severity of the injury and level of displacement, a second projection similar to the infero-superior clavicle centred over the acromioclavicular joint may be advised.
- Dependent on local protocol, subluxation of the joint may be confirmed with the patient holding a heavy weight.
- The inferior surfaces of the acromion and distal clavicle should normally be aligned.

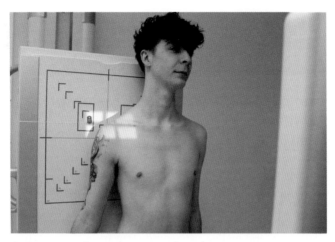

Fig. 2.3a Positioning for a right acromioclavicular joint projection.

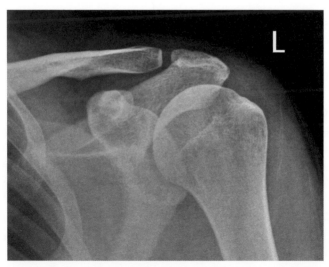

Fig. 2.3b Example of a left antero-posterior radiograph of a normal acromioclavicular joint.

ANKLE – ANTERO-POSTERIOR/ MORTISE JOINT

Position of Patient and Image Receptor (Fig. 2.4a)

- The patient is either supine or seated on the X-ray table with both legs extended and the detector placed under the affected ankle.
- A pad may be placed under the knee for comfort.
- The affected ankle may be supported in dorsiflexion by a firm 90-degree pad placed against the plantar aspect of the foot. The limb is rotated medially (approximately 20 degrees) until the medial and lateral malleoli are equidistant from the detector.
- If the patient is unable to sufficiently dorsiflex the foot, then raising the heel on a 15-degree wedge or using 5–10 degrees of cranial tube angulation can correct this problem.
- The mid-tibia may be immobilised using a sandbag.

Direction and Location of the X-ray Beam

- The collimated vertical beam is centred midway between the malleoli with the central ray at 90 degrees to an imaginary line joining the malleoli.

Essential Image Characteristics (Fig. 2.4b)

- The lower third of the tibia and fibula should be included. The inclusion of the base of fifth metatarsal is useful in trauma.
- A clear joint space between the tibia, fibula and talus should be demonstrated (commonly called the mortise view).

Additional Considerations

- If there is insufficient dorsiflexion the calcaneum will be superimposed over the lateral malleolus.

Expected DRL: ESD 0.11 mGy

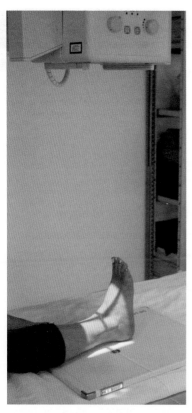

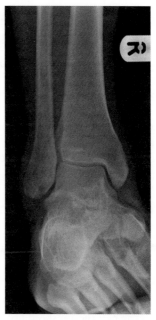

Fig. 2.4b Example of an antero-posterior ankle (mortise) radiograph.

Fig. 2.4a Positioning for an antero-posterior ankle (mortise) projection.

ANKLE – LATERAL

Position of Patient and Image Receptor (Fig. 2.5a)

- With the ankle dorsiflexed, the patient turns onto the affected side until the malleoli are superimposed vertically and the tibia is parallel to the detector.
- A 15-degree pad is placed under the lateral border of the forefoot and a pad is placed under the knee for support.

Direction and Location of the X-ray Beam

- The collimated vertical beam is centred over the medial malleolus, with the central ray at right angles to the axis of the tibia.

Essential Image Characteristics (Fig. 2.5b)

- The lower third of the tibia and fibula, base of the fifth metatarsal and the calcaneum should be included.
- The medial and lateral borders of the trochlear articular surface of the talus should be superimposed on the image.

Additional Considerations

- Over- and under-rotation lead to non-superimposition of the talar and trochlear surfaces.
- Over-rotation = fibula projected posterior to the tibia.
- Under-rotation = shaft of fibula superimposed on the tibia.
- Inversion injury of the ankle is common and may result in fracture of the lateral malleolus or the base of the fifth metatarsal. Investigation of the injury should therefore cover both areas.
- A standing lateral projection may be undertaken for conditions such as ankle arthropathy.

Expected DRL: ESD 0.12 mGy

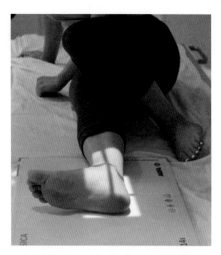

Fig. 2.5a Positioning for a lateral ankle projection.

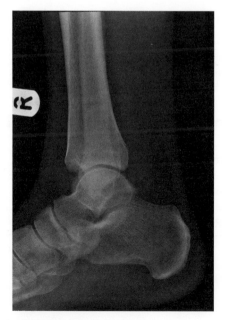

Fig. 2.5b Example of a lateral ankle radiograph.

CALCANEUM – AXIAL

Position of Patient and Image Receptor (Fig. 2.6a)

- The patient sits or lies supine on the X-ray table with both limbs extended.
- The affected leg is rotated medially until both malleoli are equidistant from the detector.
- The ankle is dorsiflexed.
- The position is maintained by using a disposable bandage or similar strapped around the forefoot and held in position by the patient.
- The detector is positioned with its lower edge just distal to the plantar aspect of the heel.

Direction and Location of the X-ray Beam

- The X-ray tube is directed cranially at an angle of 40 degrees to the plantar aspect of the heel.
- The collimated beam is centred to the plantar aspect of the heel at the level of the tubercle of the fifth metatarsal.

Essential Image Characteristics (Fig. 2.6b)

- The subtalar joint and sustentaculum tali should be visible on the axial projection.
- The inferior aspect of the calcaneum and soft tissue borders should also be demonstrated.

Expected DRL: ESD 0.2 mGy

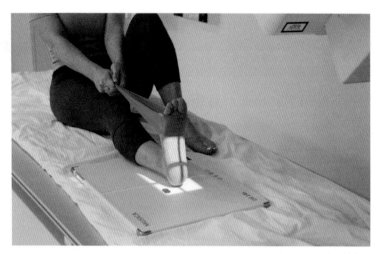

Fig. 2.6a Positioning for an axial calcaneum projection.

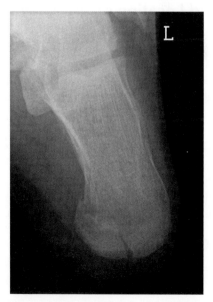

Fig. 2.6b Example of an axial calcaneum radiograph showing a fracture to the posterior aspect of the calcaneum.

CERVICAL SPINE – ANTERO-POSTERIOR C3–C7

Position of Patient and Image Receptor (Fig. 2.7a)

- The patient lies supine on the table or trolley or, if erect positioning is preferred, sits or stands with the posterior aspect of the head and shoulders against the detector in vertical position.
- The median sagittal plane is adjusted to be at right angles and to coincide with the midline of the detector.
- The neck is extended (if the patient's condition will allow) so that the lower part of the mandible is clear from the upper cervical vertebra.
- The detector is positioned to coincide with the central ray. The detector will require some cranial displacement if the tube is angled cranially.

Direction and Location of the X-ray Beam

- The collimated beam is directed with a 5–15-degree cranial angulation such that the inferior border of the symphysis menti is superimposed over the occipital bone.
- The beam is centred in the midline towards a point just below the prominence of the thyroid cartilage through the fifth cervical vertebra.

Essential Image Characteristics (Fig. 2.7b)

- The image must demonstrate the third cervical vertebra down to the cervico-thoracic junction.
- Lateral collimation should include soft tissue margins.
- The mandible should be superimposed over the occipital bone.

Additional Considerations

- A grid may be used, dependent on local protocol and patient body habitus.

Expected DRL: DAP 0.15 Gy·cm²

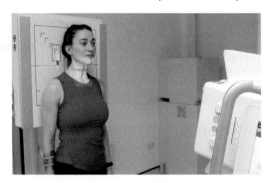

Fig. 2.7a Positioning for an antero-posterior C3–C7 cervical vertebrae projection – patient erect.

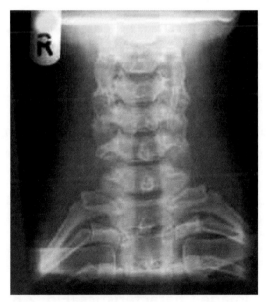

Fig. 2.7b Example of an antero-posterior cervical spine radiograph.

CERVICAL SPINE – ANTERO-POSTERIOR C1–C2 'OPEN MOUTH' (ODONTOID PEG)

Position of Patient and Image Receptor (Fig. 2.8a)

- The patient lies supine on the trolley or table or, if erect positioning is preferred, sits or stands with the posterior aspect of the head and shoulders against the detector in the vertical position.
- The medial sagittal plane is adjusted to coincide with the midline of the detector.
- The neck is extended, if possible, such that a line joining the tip of the mastoid process and the inferior border of the upper incisors is at right angles to the detector. This will superimpose the upper incisors and the occipital bone, thus allowing clear visualisation of the area of interest.
- The detector is centred at the level of the mastoid process.

Direction and Location of the X-ray Beam

- The collimated beam is directed with the perpendicular central ray along the midline to the centre of the open mouth.
- If the patient is unable to flex or extend the neck and attain the position described above, then the beam must be angled, typically 5–10 degrees cranially or caudally, to attain superimposition of the upper incisors on the occipital bone.
- The detector position will have to be altered to allow the image to be centred after beam angulation.

Essential Image Characteristics (Fig. 2.8b)

- The inferior border of the upper central incisors should be superimposed over the occipital bone.
- The whole of the articulation between the atlas and the axis must be demonstrated clearly.

- Ideally the whole of the dens, the lateral masses of the atlas and as much of the axis as possible should be included within the image.

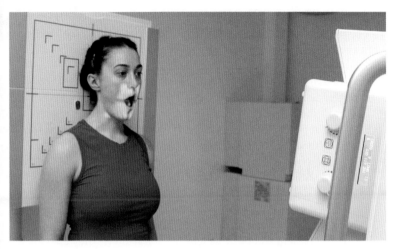

Fig. 2.8a Positioning for an antero-posterior C1–C2 cervical spine projection – patient erect.

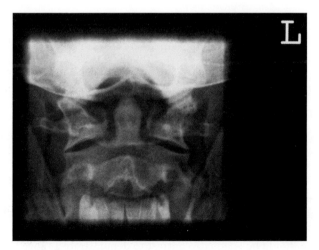

Fig. 2.8b Example of an antero-posterior C1–C2 cervical spine radiograph.

CERVICAL SPINE – LATERAL ERECT

Position of Patient and Image Receptor (Fig. 2.9a)

- The patient stands or sits with either shoulder against the detector in the vertical position. A grid may be employed dependent on local protocol and body habitus.
- The median sagittal plane should be adjusted such that it is parallel with the detector.
- The head should be extended such that the angle of the mandible is not superimposed over the cervical vertebral bodies, or the occipital bone does not obscure the posterior arch of the atlas.
- To aid immobilisation, the patient should stand with the feet slightly apart and with the shoulder resting against the detector stand.
- In order to demonstrate the lower cervical vertebra, the shoulders should be depressed. This may be achieved by asking the patient to relax their shoulders downwards. The process may be aided by asking the patient to hold a weight in each hand (if they are capable and injuries allow) and/or by making the exposure on arrested expiration.

Direction and Location of the X-ray Beam

- The collimated horizontal beam is centred over a point vertically below the mastoid process at the level of the prominence of the thyroid cartilage (C4 level).

Essential Image Characteristics (Fig. 2.9b)

- The whole of the cervical spine should be included, from the base of the skull at the foramen magnum to the superior aspect of the first thoracic vertebra.
- The mandible or occipital bone must not obscure any part of the upper vertebra.
- Angles of the mandible should be superimposed.
- Soft tissues of the neck should be included.
- There should be adequate contrast to demonstrate a range of differing densities from soft tissue to bony detail.

Expected DRL: DAP 0.15 Gy·cm²

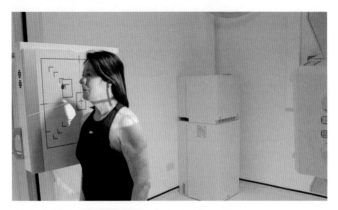

Fig. 2.9a Positioning for a lateral erect cervical spine projection.

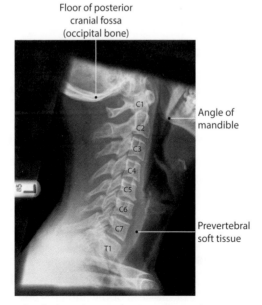

Floor of posterior cranial fossa (occipital bone)

Angle of mandible

Prevertebral soft tissue

Fig. 2.9b Example of a lateral cervical spine radiograph.

CERVICAL SPINE – LATERAL 'SWIMMERS'

Position of Patient and Image Receptor (Fig. 2.10a)

- This projection is usually carried out with the patient supine on a trauma trolley. The trolley is positioned adjacent to the vertical detector, with the patient's median sagittal plane parallel with the detector.
- The arm nearest the detector is folded over the head, with the humerus as close to the trolley top as the patient can manage. The arm and shoulder nearest the X-ray tube are depressed as far as possible.
- The shoulders are now separated vertically.
- The detector system should be raised or lowered such that the line of the vertebrae should coincide with the middle of the detector.
- This projection can also be undertaken with the patient erect, either standing or sitting, or supine.

Direction and Location of the X-ray Beam

- The collimated horizontal central ray is directed to the midline of the detector at a level just above the shoulder remote from the detector.

Essential Image Characteristics (Fig. 2.10b)

- It is imperative to ensure that the C7/T1 junction has been included on the image. It is therefore useful to include an anatomical landmark in the image, e.g. atypical second cervical vertebra. This will make it possible to count down the vertebrae and ensure that the junction has been imaged.

Additional Considerations

- Failure to ensure that the raised arm is as flat as possible against the trolley may result in the head of the humerus obscuring the region of interest.

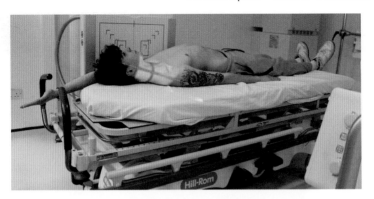

Fig. 2.10a Positioning for a lateral 'swimmers' cervical spine projection.

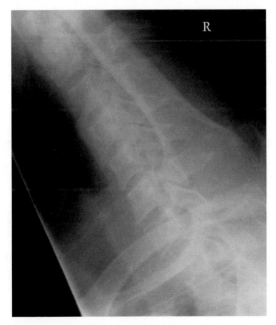

Fig. 2.10b Example of a lateral 'swimmers' cervical spine radiograph.

CERVICAL SPINE – LATERAL SUPINE

Position of Patient and Image Receptor (Fig. 2.11a)

- This projection is normally undertaken on trauma patients who arrive in the supine position, with their neck immobilised on a trolley.
- It is vitally important for the patient to depress the shoulders as much as possible (assuming no other injuries would contraindicate this).
- The detector should be vertical, with the top of the detector at the same level as the top of the ear and adjusted along with the position of the trolley to ensure that the cervical spine corresponds with the central field of the detector.
- To maximise depression of the shoulders, the exposure is taken on expiration with verbal encouragement to the patient. Alternatively authorised clinical staff can apply caudal traction to the arms to encourage shoulder distraction.

Direction and Location of the X-ray Beam

- The collimated horizontal beam is centred over a point vertically below the mastoid process at the level of the prominence of the thyroid cartilage (C4 level).

Essential Image Characteristics (Fig. 2.11b)

- See Cervical Spine – Lateral Erect.

Additional Considerations

- If the image has failed to demonstrate C7/T1 and the patient's shoulders are already depressed fully, then the application of bilateral traction will normally show half to one extra vertebra inferiorly. Additional requirement for the 'swimmers' projection or CT should be considered to demonstrate C7/T1, dependent on local protocol.

- Refer to departmental local rules for staff working in a controlled area.

Expected DRL: DAP 0.15 Gy·cm²

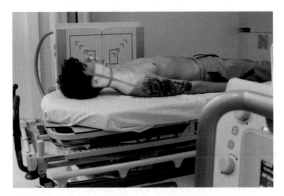

Fig. 2.11a Positioning for lateral supine cervical spine projection.

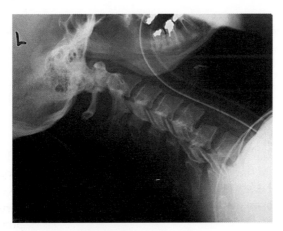

Fig. 2.11b Example of a lateral cervical spine cervical spine radiograph demonstrating fracture dislocation of C5/C6.

CERVICAL SPINE – POSTERIOR OBLIQUE

Position of Patient and Image Receptor (Fig. 2.12a)

- The patient stands or sits with the posterior aspect of their head and shoulders against the detector, with or without a grid, depending on local protocol.
- To avoid superimposition of the mandible over the spine the median sagittal plane of the trunk, including the head, is rotated through 45 degrees for the right and left sides in turn.
- The image detector is centred in the midline at the prominence of the thyroid cartilage.

Direction and Location of the X-ray Beam

- The collimated beam is angled 15 degrees cranially from the horizontal, centred to the C4/C5 junction in the centre of the soft tissue of the neck on the side nearest the tube.

Essential Image Characteristics (Fig. 2.12b)

- The intervertebral foramina should be demonstrated clearly.
- The C1–T1 vertebrae should be included within the image.
- Vertebrae should be visible without the mandible and occipital bone overlying.

Additional Considerations

- In trauma cases the projection may be undertaken with the patient supine and the beam angled 30–45 degrees to the median sagittal plane. The detector should be displaced to one side to account for the beam angulation without a grid, to avoid 'cut off'.

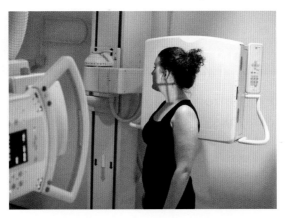

Fig. 2.12a Positioning for oblique cervical spine projection.

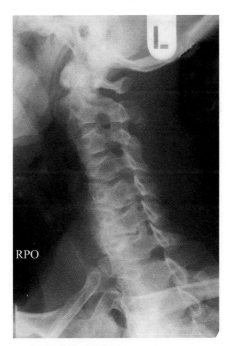

Fig. 2.12b Example of an oblique cervical spine radiograph.

93

CERVICAL SPINE – FLEXION AND EXTENSION

Position of Patient and Image Receptor (Figs. 2.13a,b)

- The patient is positioned as for the lateral projection. The patient is asked to flex the neck and to tuck the chin in towards the chest as far as is comfortably possible.
- For the second projection, the patient is asked to extend the neck by raising the chin as far as comfortably possible.
- Immobilisation can be facilitated by asking the patient to hold on to a solid object, such as the back of a chair or equipment handles.
- The central beam is centred to the detector in the mid-cervical region to ensure demonstration of the base of the skull/C1 to C7/T1.

Direction and Location of the X-ray Beam

- The collimated horizontal beam is centred over the mid-cervical region (C4).

Essential Image Characteristics (Fig. 2.13c)

- The final image should include the entire cervical vertebra, including the atlanto-occipital joints, the spinous processes and the soft tissues of the neck.

Additional Considerations

- Refer to local protocols for the need for medical supervision if undertaking these examinations on patients with suspected trauma or an unstable spine.

Expected DRL: DAP 0.15 Gy·cm^2

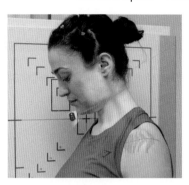

Fig. 2.13a Flexion.

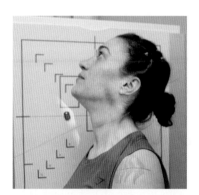

Fig. 2.13b Extension.

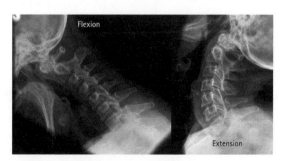

Fig. 2.13c Examples of cervical spine flexion and extension radiographs.

CHEST – POSTERO-ANTERIOR

Position of Patient and Image Receptor (Fig. 2.14a)

- Use the vertical detector with or without a grid, dependent on local protocol and body habitus. The patient should be prepared carefully, with any radio-opaque artefacts above the waist removed.
- The patient is positioned facing the detector with the chin extended and centred to the middle of the top of the detector.
- The feet are paced slightly apart so that the patient can remain steady.
- The median sagittal plane is adjusted at right angles to the middle of the detector; the shoulders are rotated forward and pressed downward in contact with the vertical detector.
- This is achieved by placing the dorsal aspect of the hands behind and below the hips with the elbows brought forward or by allowing the arms to encircle the vertical detector.

Direction and Location of the X-ray Beam

- The collimated horizontal beam is directed at right angles to the vertical detector and centred at the level of the eighth thoracic vertebra (i.e. spinous process of T7), which is coincident with the lung midpoint, found by using the level of the inferior angle of the scapula before the shoulders are rotated anteriorly.
- Exposure is made in full normal arrested inspiration.
- A focus-to-receptor distance (FRD) of 180 cm is used to minimise magnification.

Essential Image Characteristics (Fig. 2.14b)

- The lungs from above the apices to below the costo-phrenic angles should be demonstrated, with the scapulae laterally rotated and the clavicles symmetrical and equidistant from the spinous process of T4.
- Ensure sufficient inspiration so that either six ribs anteriorly or ten ribs posteriorly are visualised.

- The costo-phrenic angles, diaphragm, mediastinum, lung markings and heart should be defined sharply.

Additional Considerations

- The use of a grid for chest imaging is dependent on local protocol, positioning and patient habitus. The grid focus should be appropriate to the equipment and technique employed.

Expected DRL: DAP 0.1 Gy·cm2, ESD 0.15 mGy

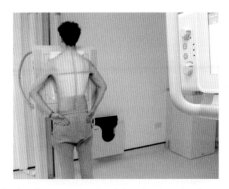

Fig. 2.14a Positioning for a postero-anterior chest projection.

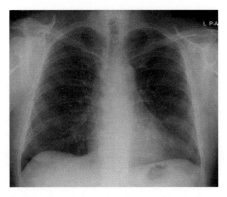

Fig. 2.14b Example of a postero-anterior chest radiograph.

CHEST – ANTERO-POSTERIOR (ERECT)

This projection is often used as an alternative when the postero-anterior projection cannot be performed due to the patient's condition. Frequently the patient is supported sitting erect on a chair or trolley.

Position of Patient and Image Receptor (Fig. 2.15a)

- The patient sits with their back against the detector secured in the vertical position, with the upper edge of the detector above the lung apices.
- The median sagittal plane is adjusted at right angles to the middle of the detector.
- Dependent on the patient's condition, the arms are extended forwards into the anatomical position and rotated internally to minimise the superimposition of the scapulae on the lung fields.

Direction and Location of the X-ray Beam

- The collimated horizontal beam is angled caudally until it is at right angles to the sternum and centred midway between the sternal notch and the xiphisternum.
- The degree of caudal angulation (5–10 degrees) for the non-kyphotic patient is dependent on patient anatomy. This will ensure maximum visualisation of the lung fields and that the clavicles do not obscure the lung apices.
- The exposure is taken on normal full inspiration.
- An FRD of at least 120 cm is essential to reduce unequal magnification of intrathoracic structures.

Essential Image Characteristics (Fig. 2.15b)

- The image should be of comparable quality to that described for the postero-anterior chest projection.

Additional Considerations

- The heart is magnified (in comparison to the postero-anterior projection) due to increased distance from the image detector, thus reducing accuracy of assessment of heart size (measured by the cardiothoracic ratio).

Expected DRL: DAP 0.15 Gy·cm2, ESD 0.2 mGy

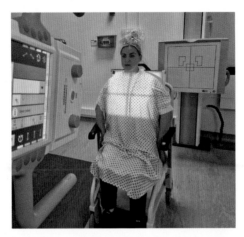

Fig. 2.15a Positioning for an antero-posterior chest projection.

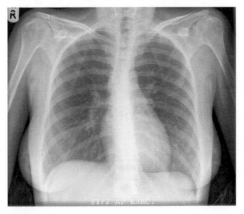

Fig. 2.15b Example of an antero-posterior chest radiograph.

CHEST – LATERAL

Position of Patient and Image Receptor (Fig. 2.16a)

- The vertical detector/Bucky system is used.
- The patient is turned to bring the side under investigation in contact with the detector.
- The median sagittal plane is adjusted parallel to the detector.
- The arms are folded over the head or raised above the head to rest on a horizontal equipment bar.
- The mid-axillary line is coincident with the middle of the detector, which is then adjusted to include the apices and the lower zones of the lungs to the level of the first lumbar vertebra.

Direction and Location of the X-ray Beam

- The collimated horizontal beam is directed at right angles to the middle of the detector coincident with the mid-axillary line.
- Exposure is made in arrested full inspiration.

Essential Image Characteristics (Fig. 2.16b)

- The image should include soft tissue superior to the apices and below the costo-phrenic angles, and the lung margins anteriorly and posteriorly.
- Image quality should be sufficient to demonstrate soft tissue detail and any pathology within the lungs and thorax.

Additional Considerations

- The projection is useful to confirm the lobular position and dimension of a lesion visualised on the initial projection, or the position of leads following pacemaker insertion.
- However, it is not a routine examination due to the additional patient dose and the increasing use of CT to examine the thorax.

Expected DRL: ESD 0.5 mGy

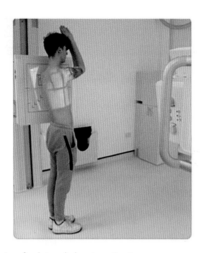

Fig. 2.16a Positioning for lateral chest projection.

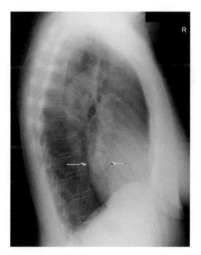

Fig. 2.16b Example of a lateral chest radiograph showing a (tumour) mass in the right (lower) middle lobe.

CHEST – SUPINE (ANTERO-POSTERIOR)

This projection is usually only utilised when the patient is unable to sit up on a bed or trolley, usually due to other injuries.

Position of Patient and Image Receptor (Fig. 2.17a)

■ With assistance, the detector is carefully positioned under the patient's chest with the upper edge of the detector above the lung apices (C7 prominence). The detector is orientated to ensure that the lung fields are included on the image.

■ The median sagittal plane is adjusted at right angles to the middle of the detector, and the patient's pelvis is checked to ensure that it is not rotated.

■ The arms are abducted from the torso laterally with the head supported on a pillow and the chin slightly raised.

Direction and Location of the X-ray Beam

■ As described for the sitting antero-posterior position except that the X-ray beam is vertical (see Chest – Antero-posterior (Erect)).

Essential Image Characteristics (Fig. 2.17b)

■ The image quality may be compromised due to the patient's condition and the drawbacks of the technique compared to the erect postero-anterior projection; i.e. accuracy of assessing cardio-thoracic ratio and assessment of conditions, as explained below. However, the apices, lateral lung margins and bases should be visualised with maximum inspiration and with no evidence of rotation.

Additional Considerations

■ There may be limited inspiration and thus loss of lung volume due to the absence of the effect of gravity on the abdominal organs, which exists in the erect position.

- Pleural effusion or haemo-/pneumothorax are optimally demonstrated on an erect image, and difficult to diagnose when the image is taken supine.
- An FRD of at least 120 cm is essential to reduce unequal magnification of intra-thoracic structures.

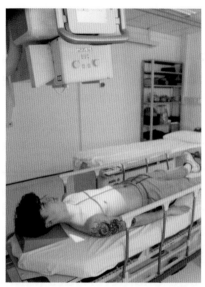

Fig. 2.17a Positioning for a supine chest (antero-posterior) projection.

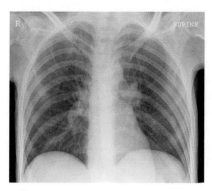

Fig. 2.17b Example of a supine chest (antero-posterior) radiograph.

CHEST – MOBILE/PORTABLE (ANTERO-POSTERIOR)

Mobile radiography should only be performed when necessary, by justifying the referral and reviewing any previous images for consistency.

Position of Patient and Image Receptor (Fig. 2.18a)

■ Where possible, the patient should be examined in an erect position; however, this may not be achievable due to the patient's condition.
■ The detector is supported behind the back of the patient, using pads or pillows, or a padded detector holder as required.
■ It is very important to minimise any rotation or lordosis, which can make interpretation difficult.

Direction and Location of the X-ray Beam

■ As described for the sitting antero-posterior position (see Chest – Antero-posterior (Erect)).

Essential Image Characteristics (Fig. 2.18b)

■ As described for the supine chest position (see Chest – Supine (Antero-posterior)).

Additional Considerations

The radiographer needs to consider issues such as:
■ correct identification of the patient;
■ moving and handling problems;
■ the need for caution when handling any patient devices such as drains or lines;
■ infection control, protective personal equipment and barrier-nursed care (see Section 1 for details);
■ radiation protection: the use of lead rubber aprons, responsibility for the controlled area and protecting patients with the use of careful technique;

- effective communication with nursing staff;
- the good practice of annotating the image with information to assist with consistency; this may include the exposure, patient position and FRD; date and time should be generated automatically.

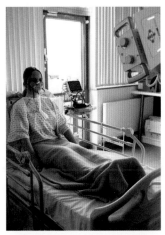

Fig. 2.18a Positioning for a mobile antero-posterior chest projection.

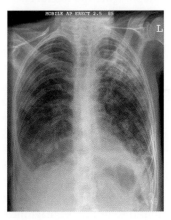

Fig. 2.18b Antero-posterior erect chest image demonstrating bilateral consolidation with a right pleural effusion due to tuberculosis.

CHEST – MOBILE (POSTERO-ANTERIOR) – PRONE

This projection is usually only utilised when the patient is being nursed in the prone position, such as for patients with COVID-19 or acute respiratory distress syndrome in the intensive care unit/intensive treatment unit.

Position of Patient and Image Receptor (Fig. 2.19a)

- The patient will generally already be placed in the prone position prior to the examination being requested.
- The wider nursing/medical team needs to be involved in the procedure to lift the patient to allow the detector to be placed and removed. This will require clear leadership, verbal instructions and several staff each side of the patient to assist with a co-ordinated lift.
- The patient is lifted often using a sheet and the detector is placed in a similar position to a postero-anterior chest X-ray, aiming to ensure the apices, diaphragms and lateral chest wall margins are included on the image.
- The median sagittal plane is adjusted at right angles to the middle of the detector, and the patient's pelvis is checked to ensure that it is not rotated.

Direction and Location of the X-ray Beam

- The beam is directed in a similar way to a postero-anterior chest X-ray, with the collimated vertical beam directed at right angles to the horizontal detector and centred at the level of the eighth thoracic vertebra (i.e. the spinous process of T7), which is coincident with the lung midpoint.
- FRD should be increased to the maximum practicable distance (120 cm as a minimum) to minimise magnification.
- If required, a small caudal angulation may be applied.
- Exposure should take place on inspiration.

piQ

Essential Image Characteristics (Fig. 2.19b)

- The image should have characteristics similar to the supine antero-posterior mobile examination.

Additional Considerations

- Take care to avoid rotation, accidental extubation of an intubated patient, movement of any lines or catheters, or injury to the patient when placing the detector.

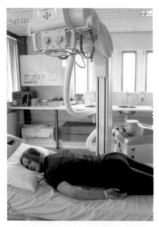

Fig. 2.19a Positioning for a mobile prone postero-anterior chest projection.

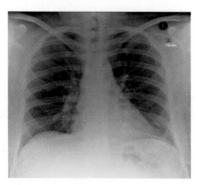

Fig. 2.19b Example of a prone postero-anterior chest radiograph.

CLAVICLE – POSTERO-ANTERIOR

Position of Patient and Image Receptor (Fig. 2.20a)

- The patient sits or stands facing a vertical detector.
- The patient's position is adjusted so that the midpoint of the clavicle is in the centre of the detector.
- The patient's head is turned away from the side being examined and the affected shoulder is rotated to ensure the affected clavicle is in close contact and parallel with the vertical detector.

Direction and Location of the X-ray Beam

- The collimated horizontal beam is centred to the midpoint of the clavicle.

Essential Image Characteristics (Fig. 2.20b)

- The clavicle, including the sterno-clavicular and acromioclavicular joints, should be included on the image.
- The clavicle should be parallel to the detector, which ensures no foreshortening of the clavicle.

Additional Considerations

- Although the clavicle is demonstrated on the antero-posterior projection, it is best practice to have the clavicle as close to the detector as possible to demonstrate optimum bony detail.
- The exposure is made on arrested respiration to minimise patient movement.

Expected DRL: ESD 0.099 mGy*

*Based on a small sample size.

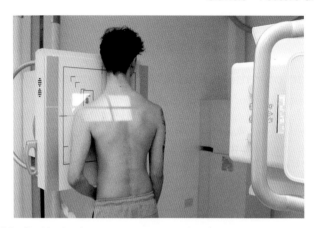

Fig. 2.20a Positioning for a postero-anterior clavicle projection.

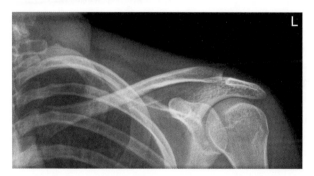

Fig. 2.20b Example of a postero-anterior clavicle radiograph.

Position of Patient and Image Receptor (Fig. 2.21a)

■ The patient sits or stands facing the X-ray tube with the affected shoulder resting against the detector. If required, angle the detector 15 degrees towards the shoulder to reduce the distortion caused by the cranially projected central beam.
■ The patient's head is turned away from the affected side.
■ The detector is displaced above the shoulder to allow the clavicle to be projected into the centre of the image, ensuring adequate presentation of anatomy and pathology.

Direction and Location of the X-ray Beam

■ The collimated horizontal beam is angled 30 degrees cranially and centred to the midpoint of the clavicle.
■ The medial aspect of the clavicle is best demonstrated by adding a 15-degree lateral angulation to the beam.

Essential Image Characteristics (Fig. 2.21b)

■ The image should demonstrate the entire length of the clavicle, including the sterno-clavicular and acromioclavicular joints.
■ The entire length of the clavicle, except for the medial end, should be projected clear of the thoracic cage.

Additional Considerations

■ The 30 degrees needed to separate the clavicle from the underlying ribs can be achieved by a combination of patient positioning and beam angulation.
■ This projection allows the clavicle to be seen from a different aspect and will often detect abnormalities not seen on the postero-anterior projection, such as discrete overriding fractures or the extent of complex fracture displacement.

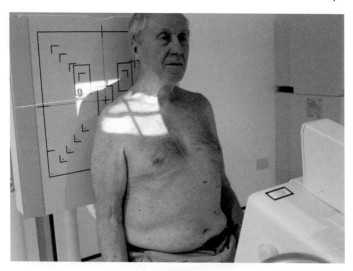

Fig. 2.21a Positioning for an infero-superior clavicle projection.

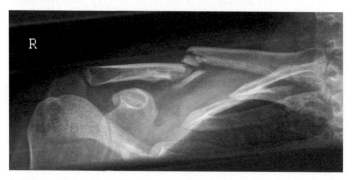

Fig. 2.21b Example of an infero-superior clavicle radiograph demonstrating a fracture.

ELBOW – ANTERO-POSTERIOR

Position of Patient and Image Receptor (Fig. 2.22a)

- The patient is seated alongside the table/detector, with the affected side nearest to the table.
- The arm is then extended fully, such that the posterior aspect of the entire limb is in contact with the detector and the palm of the hand is facing upwards.
- The detector is positioned under the elbow joint to include the distal one third of the humerus and proximal one third of the radius and ulna.
- The arm is adjusted with external rotation, such that the medial and lateral epicondyles are equidistant from the detector.
- The limb may be immobilised using sandbags.

Direction and Location of the X-ray Beam

- The collimated vertical beam is centred through the joint space 2.5 cm distal to the point midway between the medial and lateral epicondyles of the humerus.

Essential Image Characteristics (Fig. 2.22b)

- The central ray must pass through the joint space at 90 degrees to the humerus to provide a satisfactory view of the joint space.
- The image should demonstrate the distal one third of humerus and the proximal one third of the radius and ulna.

Notes

- When the patient is unable to extend the elbow to 90 degrees, a modified technique is used for the antero-posterior projection.
- If the limb cannot be moved, two projections at right angles to each other can be taken by keeping the limb in the same position and rotating the X-ray tube through 90 degrees (see the following elbow examinations for modifications).

Expected DRL: ESD 0.12 mGy

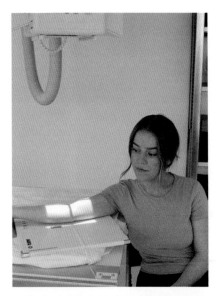

Fig. 2.22a Positioning for an antero-posterior elbow projection.

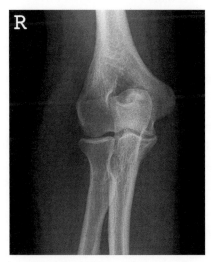

Fig. 2.22b Example of an antero-posterior elbow radiograph.

ELBOW – ALTERNATIVE ANTERO-POSTERIOR PROJECTION FOR TRAUMA

These projection may be useful if the patient is unable to extend the elbow fully. The positioning for the antero-posterior projection may be modified.

Position of Patient and Image Receptor (Figs. 2.23a–d)

This is fundamentally the same as an antero-posterior projection of the elbow and the same for all other projections; however, either the upper arm or forearm is in contact with the detector depending on the area of interest. These include:

- forearm in contact with the detector for suspected fractures of the radial head or olecranon;
- upper arm in contact with the detector for suspected supracondylar fractures;
- alternatively, the elbow remains flexed with the olecranon in contact with the detector, creating equal angles between the long axis of the bones of the forearm and the humerus with the detector;
- axial projection when the patient cannot extend their arm to any extent.

Direction and Location of the X-ray Beam

- The collimated vertical beam is centred through the joint space 2.5 cm distal to the point midway between the medial and lateral epicondyles of the humerus.

Essential Image Characteristics

- These techniques do produce some distortion of the proximal forearm and distal humerus but are used to visualise alignment and joint space.

Notes

- It is accepted that the images produced by these alternative techniques have limitations and should be used only when arm extension is not possible.

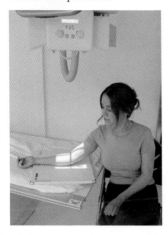

Fig. 2.23a Forearm in contact with the detector.

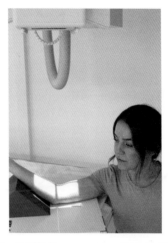

Fig. 2.23b Upper arm in contact with the detector.

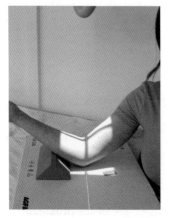

Fig. 2.23c Equal angles between the forearm and the humerus.

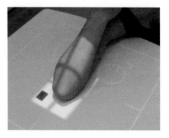

Fig. 2.23d Axial projection.

ELBOW – LATERAL

Position of Patient and Image Receptor (Fig. 2.24a)

- The patient is seated alongside the table/detector, with the affected side nearest.
- The elbow is flexed to 90 degrees and the palm of the hand is rotated so that it is at 90 degrees to the detector.
- The shoulder is lowered, or table/detector raised, so that it is at the same height as the elbow and wrist, such that the medial aspect of the entire arm is in contact with the detector.
- The detector is placed under the patient's elbow.
- The limb may be immobilised using sandbags if required.

Direction and Location of the X-ray Beam

- The vertical central ray is centred over the lateral epicondyle of the distal humerus.

Essential Image Characteristics (Fig. 2.24b)

- The central ray must pass through the joint space at 90 degrees to the humerus, i.e. the epicondyles should be superimposed.
- The image should demonstrate the distal third of humerus and the proximal third of the radius and ulna.

Notes

- Care should be taken when a supracondylar fracture of the humerus is suspected. In such cases, no attempt should be made to extend the elbow joint, and a modified technique must be employed.

Expected DRL: ESD 0.13 mGy

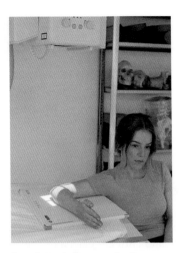

Fig. 2.24a Positioning for a lateral elbow projection.

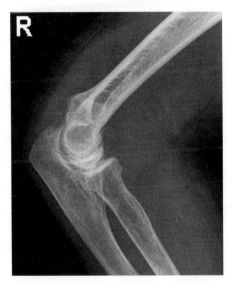

Fig. 2.24b Example of a lateral elbow radiograph with avulsion injury to the olecranon process of the olecranon-tricep tendon injury.

FACIAL BONES – OCCIPITO-MENTAL

The occipito-mental projection shows the floor of the orbits in profile, nasal region, the maxillae, inferior parts of the frontal bone and the zygomatic bone. The zygomatic arches can be seen but they appear foreshortened. The occipito-mental projection is designed to project the petrous parts of the temporal bone below the inferior part of the maxilla.

Position of Patient and Image Receptor (Fig. 2.25a)

- The projection is best performed with the patient erect, seated facing the vertical detector/Bucky.
- The patient's nose and chin are placed in contact with the midline of the Bucky/detector and then the head is adjusted to bring the orbito-meatal baseline at a 45-degree angle to the detector/Bucky.
- The horizontal central line of the detector/Bucky should be at the level of the lower orbital margins with the central exit point through the inferior nasal spine (base of the nose).
- Ensure the median sagittal plane is at right angles to the detector/ Bucky by checking the outer canthus of the eyes and the external auditory meatuses (EAMs) are equidistant.

Direction and Location of the X-ray Beam

- The collimated horizontal beam is centred to the Bucky/detector before positioning is undertaken.

Essential Image Characteristics (Fig. 2.25b)

- The petrous ridges should be demonstrated inferior to the floors of the maxillary sinuses to prove adequate angulation. There should be no rotation.

Additional Considerations

- As this is an uncomfortable position to maintain, always check the baseline angle immediately before exposure.

Notes

■ Common problems include the petrous ridges being superimposed over the inferior part of the maxillary sinuses. This demonstrates inadequate chin elevation and may be rectified by 5–10 degrees of caudal angulation on the tube, maintaining centring to the Bucky/detector.

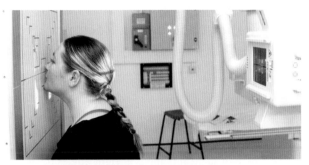

Fig. 2.25a Positioning for an occipito-mental projection.

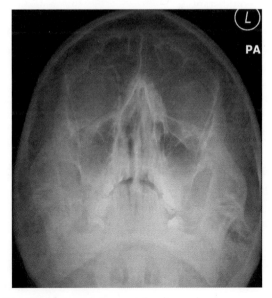

Fig. 2.25b Example of an occipito-mental radiograph.

FACIAL BONES – OCCIPITO-MENTAL 30-DEGREE CAUDAL

This projection demonstrates the lower orbital margins and the orbital floors.

Position of Patient and Image Receptor (Fig. 2.26a)

- The projection is best performed with the patient seated facing the vertical detector/Bucky.
- The patient's nose and chin are placed in contact with the midline of the Bucky/detector and then the head is adjusted to bring the orbito-meatal base line at a 45-degree angle to the Bucky/detector.
- The horizontal central line of the Bucky/detector should be at the level of the symphysis menti.
- Ensure the median sagittal plane is at right angles to the Bucky/detector by checking that the outer canthus of the eyes and the EAMs are equidistant.

Direction and Location of the X-ray Beam

- The tube is angled 30 degrees caudally from the horizontal and centred along the midline such that the central ray exits at the level of the lower orbital margins.
- To ensure the collimated beam is centred properly, the crosslines on the Bucky/detector should coincide approximately with the upper aspect of the symphysis menti region (this will vary with anatomical differences between patients).

Essential Image Characteristics (Fig. 2.26b)

- The orbital floors will be visible through the maxillary sinuses and the lower orbital margin should be clearly demonstrated. There should be no rotation.

Notes

- Common errors include failure to demonstrate the whole of the orbital floor due to under-angulation and failure to maintain the orbito-meatal baseline at 45 degrees. This may be compensated for by increasing the caudal tube angle.

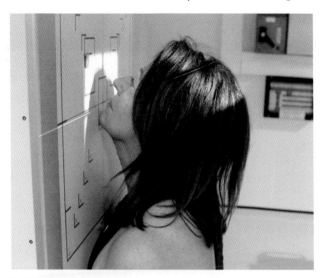

Fig. 2.26a Positioning for an occipito-mental 30-degree caudal projection.

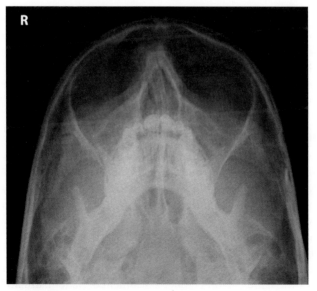

Fig. 2.26b Example of an occipito-mental 30-degree caudal radiograph.

FEMUR – ANTERO-POSTERIOR

Position of Patient and Image Receptor (Fig. 2.27a)

- The patient lies supine on the X-ray table, with both legs extended and the affected limb positioned to the centre of the table.
- The affected limb is rotated to centralise the patella over the distal femur.
- Sandbags may be applied below the knee to help maintain position.
- The Bucky/detector is located directly under the posterior aspect of the thigh to include both the hip and the knee joints.

Direction and Location of the X-ray Beam

- The collimated vertical beam is centred to the mid-shaft of the femur, with the central ray at 90 degrees to an imaginary line joining both femoral condyles.

Essential Image Characteristics (Figs. 2.27b,c)

- The length of the femur should be visualised, including the hip and knee joints. However, two images may be needed to include both joints.
- The patella should be centralised to indicate rotation has been minimised.

Additional Considerations

- In suspected fractures, the limb must not be rotated.
- The knee and hip joints should be included on the image. This may be difficult to obtain, and an additional projection of the knee or hip joint may be required if coverage is not initially achieved; however, this will depend on the referral and clinical information required.
- If the distal femur is the focus of attention, and the effects of scatter are not of pressing concern, the detector can be placed directly under the femur. Radiographer assessment of patient size and thus

the resultant scatter will determine whether a direct exposure or the use of a Bucky/grid mechanism is appropriate to produce the optimal image.

Expected DRL: ESD 1.42 mGy

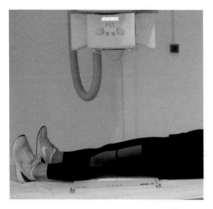

Fig. 2.27a Positioning for an antero-posterior projection of the femur – knee up.

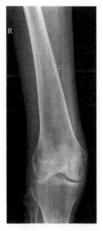

Fig. 2.27b Antero-posterior femur radiograph – knee up.

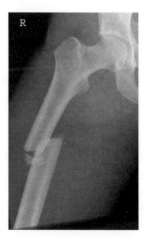

Fig. 2.27c Antero-posterior femur radiograph – hip down.

FEMUR – LATERAL

Position of Patient and Image Receptor (Fig. 2.28a)

- From the antero-posterior position, the patient rotates on to the affected side with the knee slightly flexed, and the patient is adjusted so that the femur is parallel to the table top.
- The pelvis is rotated slightly backwards to separate the upper legs, with the unaffected leg behind.
- The position of the limb is then adjusted to vertically superimpose the femoral condyles.
- Pads are used to support the opposite limb behind the one being examined.
- The Bucky/detector mechanism is located directly under the lateral aspect of the thigh to include the knee joint and as much of the femur as possible.
- Alternatively, a wireless detector is positioned directly under the thigh to include the knee and hip joints.

Direction and Location of the X-ray Beam

- The collimated vertical beam is centred to the middle of the femoral shaft, with the central ray parallel to the imaginary line joining the femoral condyles.

Essential Image Characteristics (Figs. 2.28b,c)

- The length of the femur should be visualised, including the hip and knee joints.

Additional Considerations

- Often, an additional projection of the hip joint is required if coverage is not initially achieved or the image quality is affected by scatter and/or noise in the proximal femur. However, this will depend on the clinical information required and the patient's size.

Expected DRL: ESD 1.42 mGy

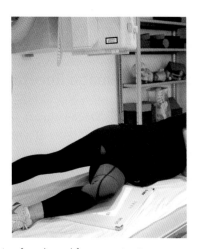

Fig. 2.28a Positioning for a lateral femur projection.

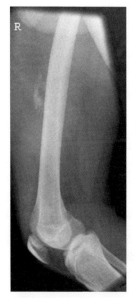

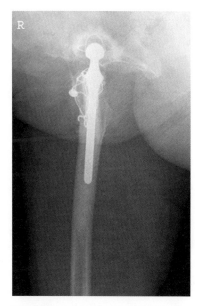

Fig. 2.28b Lateral femur radiograph – knee up.

Fig. 2.28c Lateral femur radiograph – hip down, demonstrating a hip prosthesis.

125

FINGERS – DORSI-PALMAR

Position of Patient and Image Receptor (Fig. 2.29a)

- The patient is seated alongside the table, as for a dorsi-palmar projection of the hand (see Hand – Dorsi-palmar).
- The forearm is pronated with the anterior (palmar) aspect of the finger(s) in contact with the detector.
- The finger(s) are extended and separated.
- A sandbag can be placed across the dorsal surface of the wrist for immobilisation.

Direction and Location of the X-ray Beam

- The collimated vertical beam is centred over the proximal interphalangeal joint of the affected finger.

Essential Image Characteristics (Fig. 2.29b)

- The image should include the fingertips and the distal third of the metacarpal bone, dependent on site of injury.

Additional Considerations

- It is best practice to include an adjacent uninjured finger to assist in identifying the injured digit.

Notes

- It is common practice to obtain two projections, a dorsi-palmar and a lateral.

Expected DRL: ESD 0.054 mGy

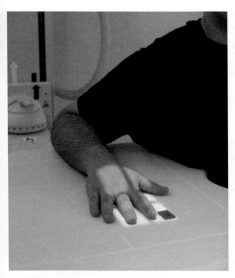

Fig. 2.29a Positioning for a dorsi-palmar finger projection.

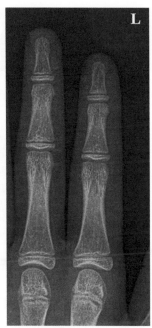

Fig. 2.29b Dorsi-palmar radiograph of the index and middle fingers – left hand.

FINGERS – LATERAL INDEX AND MIDDLE FINGERS

Position of Patient and Image Receptor (Fig. 2.30a)

- The patient is seated alongside the table with the arm abducted and medially rotated to bring the lateral aspect of the index finger into contact with the detector.
- The raised forearm is supported.
- The index finger is fully extended and the middle finger slightly flexed to avoid superimposition.
- The middle finger may be supported on a non-opaque pad.
- The remaining fingers are fully flexed into the palm of the hand and held there by the thumb.

Direction and Location of the X-ray Beam

- The collimated vertical beam is centred over the proximal inter-phalangeal joint of the affected finger.

Essential Image Characteristics (Fig. 2.30b)

- The image should include the fingertips and the distal third of the metacarpal bone, dependent on site of injury.

Additional Considerations

- Avulsion fracture of the base of the dorsal aspect of the distal phalanx is associated with injury to the insertion of the extensor digitorum tendon, leading to the mallet finger deformity.
- Avulsion fracture to the palmar aspect of the middle phalanx indicates a volar plate type of injury.
- In cases of severe trauma it may not be possible to obtain an isolated lateral projection.

Notes

■ It is common practice to obtain two projections, a dorsi-palmar and a lateral.

Expected DRL: ESD 0.054 mGy

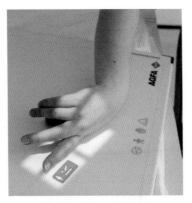

Fig. 2.30a Positioning for lateral projection of the index and middle finger.

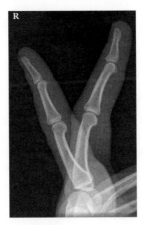

Fig. 2.30b Example of a normal lateral radiograph of the index and middle fingers.

FINGERS – LATERAL RING AND LITTLE FINGERS

Position of Patient and Image Receptor (Fig. 2.31a)

- The patient is seated alongside the table with the palm of the hand at right angles to the table and the medial aspect of the little finger in contact with the detector.
- The affected finger is extended, and the remaining fingers are fully flexed into the palm of the hand and held there by the thumb to prevent superimposition.
- It may be necessary to support the ring finger on a non-opaque pad to ensure that it is parallel to the image detector.

Direction and Location of the X-ray Beam

- The collimated vertical beam is centred over the proximal inter-phalangeal joint of the affected finger.

Essential Image Characteristics (Fig. 2.31b)

- The image should include the fingertips and the distal third of the metacarpal bone, dependent on site of injury.

Additional Considerations

- Avulsion fracture of the base of the dorsal aspect of the distal phalanx is associated with injury to the insertion of the extensor digitorum tendon, leading to the mallet finger deformity.
- Avulsion fracture to the palmar aspect of the middle phalanx indicates a volar plate type of injury.
- In cases of severe trauma, when the fingers cannot be flexed, it may be necessary to take a lateral projection of all the fingers superimposed, as for the lateral projection of the hand, but centring over the proximal interphalangeal joint of the index finger.

Notes

- It is common practice to obtain two projections, a dorsi-palmar and a lateral.

Expected DRL: ESD 0.054 mGy

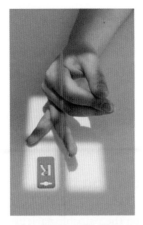

Fig. 2.31a Positioning for a lateral ring and little fingers projection.

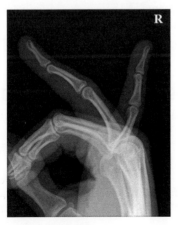

Fig. 2.31b Example of a lateral radiograph of the ring and little fingers.

FOOT – DORSI-PLANTAR

Position of Patient and Image Receptor (Fig. 2.32a)

- The patient is seated on the X-ray table supported, if necessary, with the hip and knee flexed.
- The plantar aspect of the foot is placed on the detector and the lower leg may be supported in the vertical position by the other knee.
- The detector can be raised by 15 degrees to aid positioning using a radio-opaque pad with a vertical central beam. This will improve the visualisation of the tarsal and tarso-metatarsal joints. This angulation compensates for the inclination of the longitudinal arches and reduces overshadowing of the tarsal bones.

Direction and Location of the X-ray Beam

- The collimated vertical beam is centred over the cuboid-navicular joint midway between the palpable navicular tuberosity and the tuberosity of the fifth metatarsal.
- The X-ray tube is angled 15 degrees cranially when the detector is parallel to the table.
- Alternatively, the X-ray beam can be vertical if the detector is raised by 15 degrees.

Essential Image Characteristics (Fig. 2.32b)

- The tarsal and tarso-metatarsal joints should be demonstrated when the whole foot is examined.
- Inclusion of the medial and lateral malleoli is helpful in trauma cases to exclude bony injury to these areas.

> **Expected DRL: ESD 0.075 mGy**

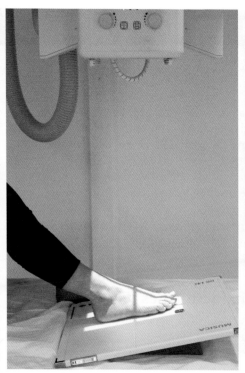

Fig. 2.32a Positioning for a dorsi-plantar foot projection with 15-degree angled pad.

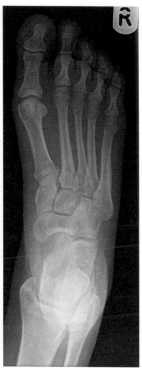

Fig. 2.32b Example of a normal dorsi-plantar foot radiograph.

FOOT – DORSI-PLANTAR OBLIQUE

Position of Patient and Image Receptor (Figs. 2.33a,b)

- From the basic dorsi-plantar position, the affected lower leg is rotated medially with the medial aspect of the foot in contact with the detector and bringing the plantar surface of the foot to approximately 30–45 degrees to the detector.
- A non-opaque angled pad may be placed under the lateral aspect of the foot to maintain the position if required.

Direction and Location of the X-ray Beam

- The collimated vertical beam is directed over the cuboid navicular joint.

Essential Image Characteristics (Fig. 2.33c)

- The dorsi-plantar oblique projection should demonstrate the inter-tarsal and tarso-metatarsal joints.
- The base of the fifth metatarsal should be demonstrated.

Additional Considerations

- Be aware of the location of possible accessory ossicles around the foot. Do not confuse these with avulsion fractures, which are generally not as rounded and well defined in appearance.
- The appearance of the unfused apophysis at the base of the fifth metatarsal in children and adolescents is variable and frequently causes confusion. (A fracture will be transverse and an apophysis will be parallel to the base of the fifth metatarsal.)

Expected DRL: ESD 0.076 mGy

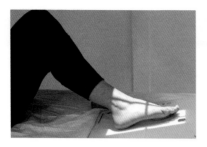

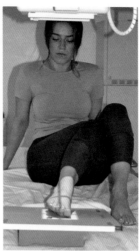

Figs. 2.33a,b Positioning for a dorsi-plantar oblique foot projection.

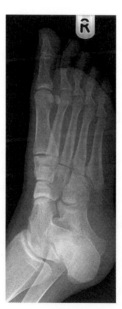

Fig. 2.33c Example of a normal dorsi-plantar oblique foot radiograph.

FOOT – LATERAL ERECT

Position of Patient and Image Receptor (Figs. 2.34a,b)

- The patient stands on a low platform with the foot being imaged placed slightly forward. The patient's weight should be on this forward foot.
- The lateral aspect of the foot is against the erect detector.
- The other foot is moved back to ensure it is not included in the image while the patient maintains their weight on the foot being imaged. Care should be taken to ensure that the hips are perpendicular to the detector.
- The image is taken in the medio-lateral position.
- To help maintain the position, the patient should rest their forearms on a convenient vertical support, e.g. the platform support mechanism.

Direction and Location of the X-ray Beam

- The collimated horizontal beam is centred to the medial aspect the foot to the base of the first metatarsal.

Essential Image Characteristics (Fig. 2.34c)

- The image should include the distal phalanges and calcaneum.
- The ankle joint and soft tissue margins of the plantar aspect of the foot should be included.
- The longitudinal arches of the foot should be clearly demonstrated.

Additional Considerations

- Frequently both feet are imaged for comparison.
- Images should be labelled as 'standing' or 'weight-bearing'.

Expected DRL: ESD 0.092 mGy

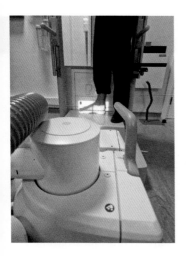
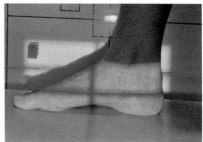

Figs. 2.34a,b Positioning for lateral erect foot projection.

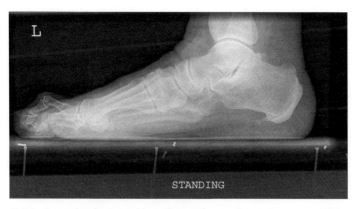

Fig. 2.34c Example of a normal lateral erect foot radiograph.

FOREARM – ANTERO-POSTERIOR

Position of Patient and Image Receptor (Fig. 2.35a)

- The patient is seated alongside the table, with the affected side nearest to it.
- The arm is abducted, and the elbow joint is fully extended, with the supinated forearm resting on the table.
- The shoulder is lowered to the same level as the elbow joint, or the detector is raised.
- The detector is placed under the forearm to include the wrist joint and the elbow joint.
- The arm is adjusted such that the radial and ulnar styloid processes and the medial and lateral epicondyles are equidistant from the detector.
- The lower end of the humerus and the hand may be immobilised using sandbags.

Direction and Location of the X-ray Beam

- The collimated vertical beam is centred to the midline of the forearm to a point midway between the wrist and elbow joint.

Essential Image Characteristics (Fig. 2.35b)

- Both the elbow and the wrist joint must be demonstrated on the radiograph.
- Both joints should be seen in the true antero-posterior position, with the radial and ulnar styloid processes and the epicondyles of the humerus equidistant from the detector.

Notes

- When the patient is unable to extend the elbow to 90 degrees, a modified technique is used for the antero-posterior projection.
- If the limb cannot be moved, two projections at right angles to each other can be taken by keeping the limb in the same position and rotating the X-ray tube accordingly to attain two projections at 90 degrees to each other.

- The postero-anterior projection of the forearm with the wrist pronated is not diagnostic because, in this projection, the radius is superimposed over the ulna for part of its length.

Expected DRL: ESD 0.13 mGy

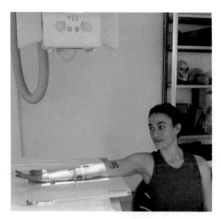

Fig. 2.35a Positioning for an antero-posterior forearm projection.

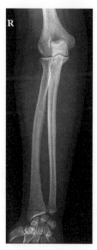

Fig. 2.35b Example of an antero-posterior forearm radiograph.

FOREARM – LATERAL

Position of Patient and Image Receptor (Fig. 2.36a)

- From the antero-posterior position, the elbow is flexed to 90 degrees.
- The humerus is rotated internally to 90 degrees to bring the medial aspect of the upper arm, elbow, forearm, wrist and hand into contact with the table/detector.
- The detector is placed under the forearm to include the wrist and elbow joint.
- The arm is adjusted such that the radial and ulnar styloid processes and the medial and lateral epicondyles are superimposed.
- The lower end of the humerus and the hand can be immobilised using sandbags.

Direction and Location of the X-ray Beam

- The collimated vertical beam is centred in the midline of the forearm to a point midway between the wrist and elbow joints.

Essential Image Characteristics (Fig. 2.36b)

- Both the elbow and the wrist joint must be demonstrated on the image.
- Both joints should be seen in the true lateral position, with the radial and ulnar styloid processes and the epicondyles of the humerus superimposed.

Notes

- In trauma cases, it may not be possible to move the arm into the position described, and a modified technique may need to be employed to ensure that diagnostic images are obtained.
- If the limb cannot be moved through 90 degrees, then a horizontal beam should be used.
- Both joints should be included on each image.

Expected DRL: ESD 0.13 mGy

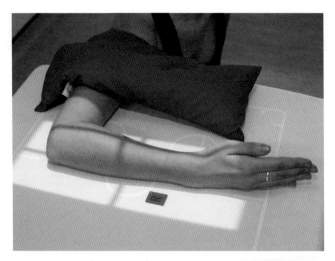

Fig. 2.36a Positioning for a lateral forearm projection.

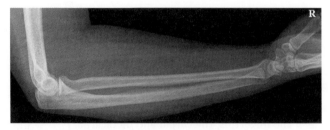

Fig. 2.36b Example of a lateral forearm radiograph.

HAND – DORSI-PALMAR

Position of Patient and Image Receptor (Fig. 2.37a)

- The patient is seated alongside the table/detector with the affected arm nearest to the table.
- The forearm is pronated and placed on the table with the palmar surface of the hand in contact with the detector.
- The fingers are separated and extended but relaxed to ensure that they remain in contact with the detector.
- The wrist is adjusted so that the radial and ulna styloid processes are equidistant from the detector.
- A sandbag may be placed over the lower forearm for immobilisation.

Direction and Location of the X-ray Beam

- The collimated vertical beam is centred over the head of the third metacarpal.

Essential Image Characteristics (Fig. 2.37b)

- The image should demonstrate all the phalanges, including the soft tissue of the fingertips, the carpal and metacarpal bones, and the distal end of the radius and ulna.
- The interphalangeal and metacarpo-phalangeal and carpo-meta-carpal joints should be demonstrated.

Notes

- It is common practice to obtain a minimum of two projections, a dorsi-palmar and an oblique. If a dislocation or displaced fracture is demonstrated then a lateral projection is also required.

> **Expected DRL: ESD 0.058 mGy**

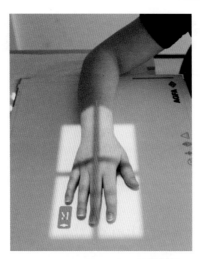

Fig. 2.37a Positioning for a dorsi-palmar hand projection.

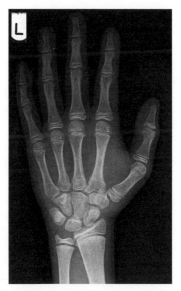

Fig. 2.37b Example of a dorsi-palmar hand radiograph.

HAND – DORSI-PALMAR OBLIQUE

Position of Patient and Image Receptor (Fig. 2.38a)

- From the basic dorsi-palmar position, the hand is rotated externally 45 degrees with the fingers parallel to the detector.
- The fingers should be separated slightly, and the hand may be supported on a 45-degree non-opaque pad.
- A sandbag may be placed over the distal forearm for immobilisation.

Direction and Location of the X-ray Beam

- The collimated vertical beam is centred to the head of the second metacarpal.

Essential Image Characteristics (Fig. 2.38b)

- The image should demonstrate all the phalanges, including the soft tissue adjacent to the distal phalanx, the carpal and metacarpal bones, and the distal end of the radius and ulna.
- The heads of the metacarpals should not be superimposed.

Expected DRL: ESD 0.06 mGy

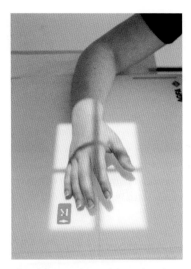

Fig. 2.38a Positioning for a dorsi-palmar oblique hand projection.

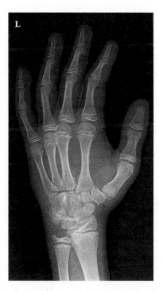

Fig. 2.38b Example of a dorsi-palmar oblique hand radiograph.

HAND – LATERAL

Position of Patient and Image Receptor (Fig. 2.39a)

- From the dorsi-palmar position, the hand is rotated externally by 90 degrees.
- The palm of the hand is perpendicular to the detector, with the fingers extended and the thumb abducted parallel to the detector and supported on a non-opaque pad if required.
- The metacarpals and carpal bones, and radial and ulnar styloid processes are superimposed.

Direction and Location of the X-ray Beam

- The collimated vertical beam is centred over the head of the second metacarpal.

Essential Image Characteristics (Fig. 2.39b)

- Common fifth metacarpal fractures are easily identified but the lateral projection allows demonstration of displacement or angulation.
- Diagnosis of fractures and/or dislocation at the carpo-metacarpal joints is limited by under- or over-rotation.

Notes

- If the projection is undertaken to identify the position of a foreign body, the exposure should be optimised to demonstrate the soft tissue with a marker identifying the site of entry of the foreign body.

Expected DRL: ESD 0.081 mGy

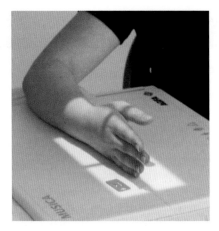

Fig. 2.39a Positioning for a lateral hand projection.

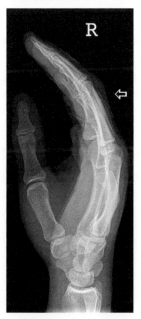

Fig. 2.39b Example of a lateral hand radiograph demonstrating a foreign body marker and healed fracture to the fifth metacarpal.

147

Position of Patient and Image Receptor (Fig. 2.40a)

- The patient is positioned as described for the basic pelvis and basic bilateral hip projections (see Pelvis – Antero-posterior).
- To avoid pelvic rotation the anterior superior iliac spines must be equidistant from the X-ray table top or erect Bucky mechanism if the examination is undertaken erect.
- The affected limb is internally rotated to bring the femoral neck parallel to the table top, supported by sandbags if necessary.
- In certain clinical circumstances, an orthopaedic templating ball bearing may be used. When placed, this ball bearing is generally positioned in the groin area, approximately level with the greater trochanter to ensure equivalent magnification of the ball bearing and the bony anatomy.

Direction and Location of the X-ray Beam

- The collimated vertical beam is centred 2.5 cm distally along the perpendicular bisector of a line joining the anterior superior iliac spine and the symphysis pubis, over the femoral pulse.
- The primary beam should be collimated to the area under examination.

Essential Image Characteristics (Fig. 2.40b)

- The acetabular floor, greater trochanter and proximal femur 2.5 cm below the lesser trochanter should be demonstrated, with the femoral neck in profile.
- The image must include the proximal third of the femur. When the examination is undertaken to show the positioning and integrity of an arthroplasty the whole length of the prosthesis, including the femur inferior to the cement, must be visualised.

Notes

- Over-rotating the limb internally will bring the greater trochanter into profile. This may be a useful supplementary projection for a suspected avulsion fracture to this bone.

Expected DRL: ESD 2.83 mGy

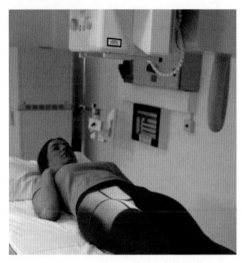

Fig. 2.40a Positioning for an antero-posterior single hip joint projection.

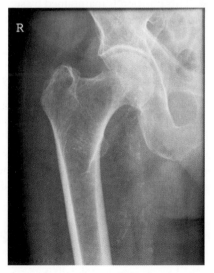

Fig. 2.40b Example of an antero-posterior single hip radiograph.

HIP – LATERAL AIR-GAP TECHNIQUE (TRAUMA)

This technique is used routinely in all patients with a suspected femoral neck fracture. A detector in the vertical Bucky is usually used with a grid (dependent on equipment and local protocol). This technique produces an image with improved resolution due to the reduction in scattered radiation incident upon the detector in comparison to standard horizontal beam lateral.

Position of Patient and Image Receptor (Figs. 2.41a,b)

- The patient lies supine on the trolley with the pelvis adjusted to ensure there is no rotation. If the patient is very slender it may be necessary to place a non-opaque pad under the buttocks so that the whole of the affected hip can be included in the image.
- The unaffected limb is then raised until the thigh is vertical, with the knee flexed. This position is maintained by supporting the lower leg on a stool or specialised equipment. The trolley is rotated to an angle of approximately 45 degrees to bring the longitudinal axis of the affected femoral neck parallel to the detector.
- The tube is positioned with an FRD of 150 cm to compensate for the increased object-to-receptor distance (ORD) due to the patient's rotation.

Direction and Location of the X-ray Beam

- The collimated horizontal beam is centred through the affected groin at the position of the groin crease with the central ray directed horizontally and at right angles to the detector and collimated closely to the area to improve the image contrast.

Essential Image Characteristics (Fig. 2.41c)

- The image should be of diagnostic quality with resolution and contrast to optimally demonstrate fine detail. As with the horizontal

beam lateral examination (see Hip – Lateral Neck of Femur) the femoral neck is optimally demonstrated with no foreshortening.
■ Careful technique and close collimation will assist in reducing the patient dose.

Expected DRL: ESD 8.12 mGy

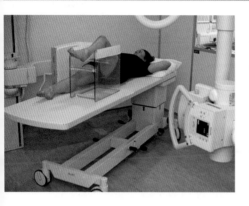
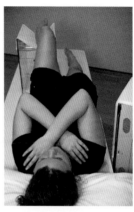

Figs. 2.41a,b Positioning for a lateral neck of femur projection using the air-gap technique.

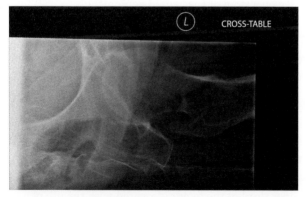

Fig. 2.41c Example of a lateral neck of femur radiograph using the air-gap technique, demonstrating high resolution.

HIP – LATERAL NECK OF FEMUR

This projection is used as an alternative projection to the lateral air-gap technique. It can be undertaken on an imaging table or with the patient remaining on a trauma trolley when it is not possible to move the patient.

Position of Patient and Image Receptor (Fig. 2.42a)

- The patient lies supine on the trolley or X-ray table with their legs extended and the pelvis adjusted to ensure the median sagittal plane is perpendicular to the table top. If the patient is very slender it may be necessary to place a non-opaque pad under the buttocks so that the whole of the affected hip can be included in the image.
- The detector is positioned vertically and the shorter edge pressed firmly against the waist, just above the iliac crest. The longitudinal axis of the detector should be parallel to the neck of the femur. This can be approximated by placing a 45-degree foam pad between the front of the detector and the lateral aspect of the pelvis.
- The unaffected limb is then raised until the thigh is vertical, with the knee flexed. This position is maintained by supporting the lower leg on a stool or specialised equipment.

Direction and Location of the X-ray Beam

- The collimated horizontal beam is centred through the affected groin midway between the femoral pulse and the palpable prominence of the greater trochanter, with the central ray directed horizontally and at right angles to the detector. It should be collimated closely to the area to improve the image contrast.

Essential Image Characteristics (Fig. 2.42b)

- A high-quality image of the acetabulum, femoral neck, trochanters and upper third of the femur is assured with the use of a stationary grid and minimal ORD.

Notes

- A relatively high kV is necessary (e.g. 100 kV) to penetrate the thigh without overexposing the trochanteric region. It is essential to ensure the detector is perpendicular to the central X-ray beam to exclude 'grid cut-off'.

Expected DRL: ESD 8.12 mGy

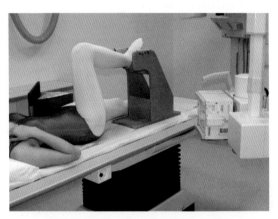

Fig. 2.42a Positioning for a lateral neck of femur projection.

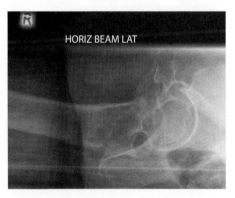

HORIZ BEAM LAT

Fig. 2.42b Example of a lateral neck of femur radiograph showing subcapital fracture.

HIP – POSTERIOR OBLIQUE (LAUENSTEIN'S)

This examination is undertaken on a non-fractured hip under examination for the hip joint (rather than the femoral neck).

Position of Patient and Image Receptor (Fig. 2.43a)

- The patient lies supine on the X-ray table, legs extended. The median sagittal plane coincides with the long axis of the X-ray table Bucky system.
- The patient rotates through 45 degrees onto the affected side with the hip abducted 45 degrees and flexed 45 degrees and is supported in this position by non-opaque pads.
- The knee is flexed to bring the lateral aspect of the thigh in contact with the table top and the knee rests on the table in the lateral position with the opposite limb raised and supported.
- The detector is centred at the level of the femoral pulse in the groin and should include the proximal third of femur. The upper border of the detector should be level with the anterior superior iliac spine.

Direction and Location of the X-ray Beam

- The collimated vertical beam is centred to the femoral pulse in the groin of the affected side, with the central ray perpendicular to the detector.
- The long axis of the primary beam is adjusted by turning the light beam diaphragm to coincide with the long axis of the femur.
- The primary beam needs to be collimated to the area under examination.

Essential Image Characteristics (Fig. 2.43b)

- This projection is not used to demonstrate the neck of the femur and should not be used as a first-line projection for a suspected fracture in this region.
- Used in conjunction with the antero-posterior projection it shows the satisfactory position of internal fixation pins and plates.

Notes

- If the unaffected side is raised greater than 45 degrees the superior pubic ramus may be superimposed on the acetabulum.
- The patient requires a degree of mobility to be positioned satisfactorily and should not experience any great discomfort in maintaining the position.

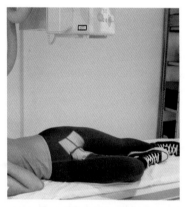

Fig. 2.43a Positioning for a posterior oblique hip joint projection.

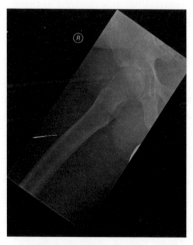

Fig. 2.43b Example of a posterior oblique hip joint radiograph.

HIPS (BOTH) – LATERAL ('FROG'S LEGS POSITION')

Position of Patient and Image Receptor (Fig. 2.44a)

- The patient lies supine on the X-ray table with the anterior superior iliac spines equidistant from the table top to avoid rotation of the pelvis.
- The median sagittal plane is perpendicular to the table and coincides with the centre of the table and Bucky/detector mechanism.
- The hips and knees are flexed and both limbs rotated laterally through approximately 60 degrees. This movement separates the knees and brings the plantar aspect of the feet in contact with each other.
- The limbs are supported in this position by pads and sandbags.
- The image detector is centred at the level of the femoral pulse in landscape orientation, to include both hip joints.

Direction and Location of the X-ray Beam

- The collimated vertical beam is centred in the midline at the level of the femoral pulse with the central ray perpendicular to the detector.

Essential Image Characteristics (Fig. 2.44b)

- The examination is undertaken to allow comparison of both hip joints and femoral head epiphyses in paediatric patients, and therefore the external hip rotation should be equal to allow this.

Notes

- A lateral rotation of 60 degrees demonstrates the hip joints.
- A modified technique with the limbs rotated laterally through 15 degrees and the plantar aspect of the feet in contact with the table top demonstrates the neck of the femur.
- If the patient is unable to achieve 60-degree rotation, it is important to apply the same degree of rotation to both limbs without losing symmetry.

- In very young children a Bucky grid is not required. The child may be placed directly onto the detector.

Expected DRL: DAP 2.2 Gy·cm², ESD 4 mGy (adult)

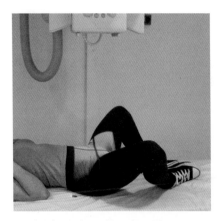

Fig. 2.44a Positioning for 'frog's legs' lateral projection.

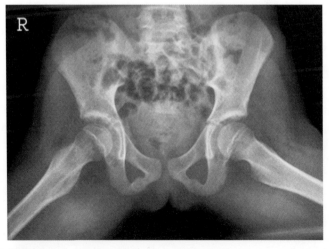

Fig. 2.44b Example of a normal paediatric radiograph demonstrating both hips in lateral projection ('frog's legs').

HUMERUS – ANTERO-POSTERIOR

Position of Patient and Image Receptor (Fig. 2.45a)

- Generally, the examination is conducted with the patient sitting or standing with their back in contact with a vertical image detector.
- The patient is rotated towards the affected side to bring the posterior aspect of the shoulder, upper arm and elbow into contact with the image detector.
- The position of the patient is adjusted to ensure that the medial and lateral epicondyles of the humerus are equidistant from the image detector.
- If the patient is unable to stand or sit upright, then supine imaging can allow greater stability for the examination.

Direction and Location of the X-ray Beam

- The collimated horizontal beam is directed at right angles to the shaft of the humerus and centred midway between the shoulder and elbow joint.

Essential Image Characteristics (Fig. 2.45b)

- The exposure should be adjusted to ensure that the area of interest is clearly visualised.

Notes

- A type of injury commonly found in children is a fracture of the lower end of the humerus just proximal to the condyles (a supracondylar fracture). The injury is very painful and even small movements of the limb can exacerbate the injury, causing further damage to adjacent nerves and blood vessels.
- Any supporting sling should not be removed, and the patient should not be asked to extend the elbow joint or to rotate the arm or forearm.
- It is common practice to obtain two projections; antero-posterior and lateral.

Expected DRL: ESD 0.28 mGy

Humerus – Antero-posterior

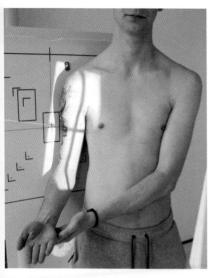

Fig. 2.45a Positioning for an antero-posterior humerus projection.

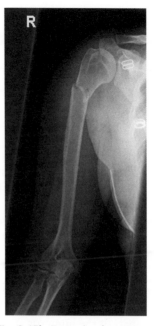

Fig. 2.45b Example of an antero-posterior radiograph of the right humerus showing a fracture of the proximal shaft of the humerus (note a bra artefact).

HUMERUS – LATERAL

Position of Patient and Image Receptor (Fig. 2.46a)

- As with the antero-posterior projection, the lateral projection is generally obtained in the erect position, but if adaption is required the projection can be obtained in a supine or semi-erect position on a bed or trolley.
- From the anterior position, the patient is rotated through 180 degrees until the antero-lateral aspect of the injured arm is in contact with the image detector, with the arm moved away from the trunk of the body.
- The patient's arm is now abducted and rotated further until the arm is just clear of the rib cage but still in contact with the image detector.

Direction and Location of the X-ray Beam

- The collimated horizontal beam is directed at right angles to the shaft of the humerus and centred midway between the shoulder and elbow joint.

Essential Image Characteristics (Fig. 2.46b)

- The exposure should be adjusted to ensure that the area of interest is clearly visualised. This should include the glenohumeral and acromioclavicular joint areas proximally and the elbow joint and proximal quarter of the radius and ulna distally.

Notes

- The patient should be made as comfortable as possible to assist in immobilisation.
- The X-ray beam should be collimated carefully to ensure that the primary beam does not extend beyond the area of the detector.

Expected DRL: ESD 0.35 mGy

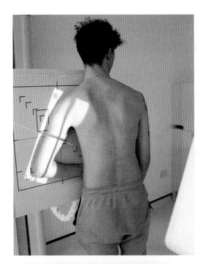

Fig. 2.46a Positioning for a lateral humerus projection.

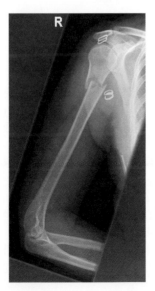

Fig. 2.46b Example of a lateral humerus radiograph showing a fracture of the proximal shaft of the humerus (note a bra artefact).

KNEE – ANTERO-POSTERIOR

Position of Patient and Image Receptor (Figs. 2.47a,b)

- This projection can be obtained in the weight-bearing (erect) or supine (conventional) position.
- Weight-bearing (erect) positioning is increasingly obtained as the first-line projection, unless the patient is unable to safely stand or if there has been recent trauma.
- Erect: the patient stands with their back against the vertical detector (grid removed), using it for support if necessary. The patient's weight is distributed equally.
- Supine: the patient is supine or seated on the table or trolley (e.g. in trauma cases) with both limbs extended. The detector is positioned behind the knee joint.
- The knee is rotated so that the patella lies equally between the femoral condyles.
- The centre of the detector is level with the palpable upper borders of the tibial condyles.
- Depending on local protocol, a measuring device, such as an orthopaedic templating ball bearing, may be placed adjacent to the joint, at the level of the intercondylar eminence, to allow accurate planning of the correct size for any potential joint prosthesis.

Direction and Location of the X-ray Beam

- The collimated horizontal beam is centred 1 cm below the apex of the patella through the joint space, with the central ray at 90 degrees to the long axis of the tibia (midway between the palpable upper borders of the tibial condyles).
- Occasionally, both knees are requested for comparison, in which case both knees can often be imaged at the same time with the beam centred at a point midway between both knees at a level 1 cm below both patellae.

Essential Image Characteristics (Fig. 2.47c)

- The patella must be centralised over the distal femoral condyles by internally rotating the foot and lower leg.
- The image should include the proximal third of the tibia and fibula and distal third of the femur.

> **Expected DRL: ESD 0.3 mGy**

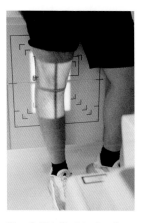

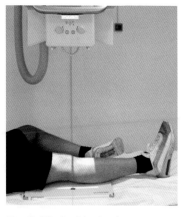

Fig. 2.47a Positioning for an antero-posterior standing erect knee projection.

Fig. 2.47b Positioning for an antero-posterior supine knee projection.

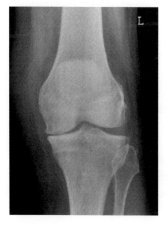

Fig. 2.47c Example of an erect antero-posterior knee radiograph with degenerative changes.

KNEE – LATERAL (BASIC)

Position of Patient and Image Receptor (Fig. 2.48a)

- The patient lies on the side to be examined, with the knee flexed at 45 degrees (i.e. 135 degrees from back of calf to back of the thigh).
- The other limb is brought forward in front of the one being examined and supported on a sandbag.
- A sandbag may be placed under the ankle of the affected side to bring the long axis of the tibia parallel to the detector. Dorsiflexion of the foot helps maintain this position.
- The position of the limb is now adjusted to ensure that the femoral condyles are superimposed vertically.
- The medial tibial condyle is placed level with the centre of the detector.

Direction and Location of the X-ray Beam

- The collimated vertical beam is centred to the middle of the superior border of the medial tibial condyle, with the central ray at 90 degrees to the long axis of the tibia.

Essential Image Characteristics (Fig. 2.48b)

- The patella should be projected clear of the femur.
- The femoral condyles should be superimposed.
- The proximal tibio-fibular joint is not clearly visible. (Approximately one third of the fibula head should be superimposed behind the tibia.)

Additional Considerations

- A small cranial tube angulation of 5–7 degrees can help superimpose the femoral condyles.
- Over-rotation = fibula is projected too posteriorly.
- Under-rotation = fibula head is hidden behind the tibia.
- Identification of the adductor tubercle indicates the medial femoral condyle and can help the radiographer to correct positioning faults.

■ This projection may also be acquired in the weight-bearing position against a vertical detector.

Expected DRL: ESD 0.3 mGy

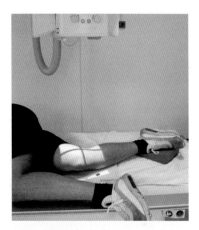

Fig. 2.48a Positioning for a lateral knee (basic) projection.

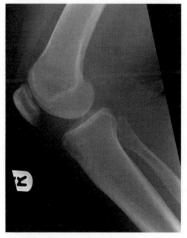

Fig. 2.48b Example of a lateral knee radiograph.

KNEE – HORIZONTAL BEAM LATERAL (TRAUMA)

There are two potential methods for this projection: the medio-lateral technique and the latero-medial technique. The latero-medial method is used in trauma cases when the patient is unable to undertake the positioning required. The medio-lateral method is technically better as it helps superimpose the femoral condyles.

The latero-medial technique is described below.

Position of Patient and Image Receptor (Figs. 2.49a,b)

- The patient remains on the trolley or bed, with the limb gently raised and supported on pads.
- If possible, the leg may be rotated slightly to centralise the patella between the femoral condyles.
- The imaging detector is supported vertically against the medial aspect of the knee with its centre at the level of the upper border of the tibial condyle.
- The positioning method for the medio-lateral is shown in Fig. 2.48b with the unaffected leg positioned over the side of the table. Alternatively the patient elevates the unaffected leg using a leg support similar for that used for a lateral horizontal hip projection (Fig. 2.41a).

Direction and Location of the X-ray Beam

- The collimated horizontal beam is centred to the upper border of the lateral tibial condyle, at 90 degrees to the long axis of the tibia with the X-ray tube angled caudally 3–5 degrees.

Essential Image Characteristics (Fig. 2.49c)

- The image should demonstrate the lower one third of the femur and proximal one third of the tibia. The femoral condyles should be superimposed, and the soft tissues adequately demonstrated to visualise any fluid levels within the suprapatellar pouch.

Additional Considerations

- This projection replaces the conventional lateral one in all cases of injury including suspected fracture of the patella.
- No attempt must be made to either flex or extend the knee joint as this may result in fragments of a transverse patellar fracture being separated by the opposing muscle pull.
- Any rotation of the limb must be from the hip, with support given to the whole leg.
- By using a horizontal beam, a lipohaemarthrosis may be visualised. This is a fat/fluid level which is caused by an intra-articular fracture leaking fat and blood from the bone marrow into the joint.

Expected DRL: ESD 0.3 mGy

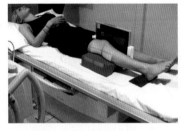

Fig. 2.49a Positioning for a horizontal beam latero-medial knee projection.

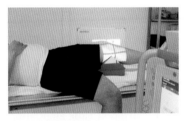

Fig. 2.49b Positioning for a horizontal beam medio-lateral knee projection.

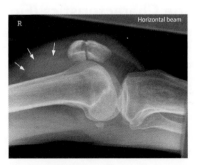

Fig. 2.49c Example of a horizontal beam knee radiograph showing a fracture of the patella with joint effusion and lipohaemarthrosis in the suprapatellar bursa (arrows).

KNEE – TUNNEL/INTERCONDYLAR NOTCH

Position of Patient and Image Receptor (Fig. 2.50a)

- The patient is either supine or seated on the X-ray table, with the affected knee flexed to approximately 60 degrees.
- A suitable pad is placed under the knee to help maintain the position.
- The limb is rotated to centralise the patella over the distal femur.
- The image detector is placed on top of the pad as close as possible to the posterior aspect of the knee and displaced towards the femur. When using a large detector this needs to be placed with the upper edge adjacent to the mid to upper femoral region posteriorly.

Direction and Location of the X-ray Beam

- The collimated beam is centred immediately below the apex of the patella.
- Two different tube angulations are used in relation to the long axis of the tibia: 90 degrees = posterior aspect of the notch is shown; 100 degrees = anterior aspect of the notch is shown.

Essential Image Characteristics (Figs. 2.50b,c)

- The lower femur and upper tibia are included, with the intercondylar notch clearly seen, which should demonstrate any radio-opaque loose bodies.

Additional Considerations

- Commonly only the 90-degree angulation is used.
- Take care when flexing the knee if a fracture is suspected.
- An alternative projection to obtain similar diagnostic information is the postero-anterior ('racing start') projection, which can be used in fitter patients who can tolerate the kneeling position.

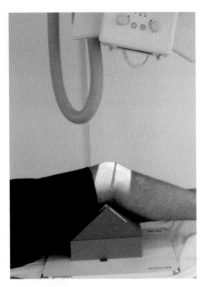

Fig. 2.50a Positioning for the intercondylar projection using either a 90- or 110-degree beam angulation to the tibia.

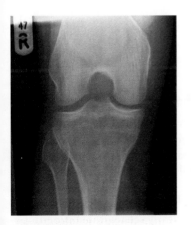

Fig. 2.50b Intercondylar image 90-degree angulation.

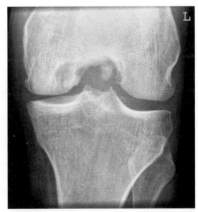

Fig. 2.50c Intercondylar image 110-degree angulation, showing a loose body.

KNEE – 'SKYLINE' PATELLAR (SUPERO-INFERIOR)

There are a number of methods of achieving the skyline projection, including:

- supero-inferior – beam directed downwards;
- infero-superior – patient supine; knee flexed with detector held vertically in a detector holder and beam directed horizontally;
- infero-superior – patient prone.

The supero-inferior method described has the advantage that the radiation beam is not directed at the gonads.

This method describes using the detector placed in a horizontal position with the patient sat on a chair or edge of the table with the knee overhanging the detector as described below.

Position of Patient and Image Receptor (Fig. 2.51a)

- The patient sits on the X-ray table with the affected knee flexed over the side.
- Ideally, the leg should be flexed to 45 degrees from full extension; however, some referrers may request skyline projections with a specified amount of flexion, for example 20 degrees. Too much flexion reduces the retro-patellar spacing.
- The detector is supported horizontally on a stool at the level of the inferior tibial tuberosity border.

Direction and Location of the X-ray Beam

- The collimated vertical central beam is centred over the posterior aspect of the proximal border of the patella. The central ray should be parallel to the long axis of the patella.
- The beam is collimated to the patella and femoral condyles.

Essential Image Characteristics (Fig. 2.51b)

- The retro-patellar space should be clearly seen without superimposition of the femur or tibia within the patella-femoral joint.
- Not enough flexion will cause the tibial tuberosity to overshadow the retro-patellar joint.

- Too much flexion will cause the patella to track over the lateral femoral condyle.

Additional Considerations

- There are at least three methods of achieving the skyline patella projection; however, the supero-inferior method is reasonably quick and has radiation protection advantages.

Expected DRL: ESD 0.28 mGy

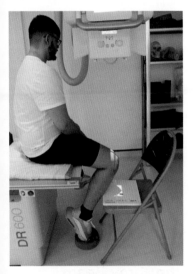

Fig. 2.51a Positioning for a skyline (supero-inferior) patellar projection.

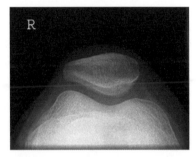

Fig. 2.51b Example of a normal skyline patellar radiograph.

LUMBAR SPINE – ANTERO-POSTERIOR

Position of Patient and Image Receptor (Fig. 2.52a)

- This projection can be obtained supine or against a vertical detector. The method below describes the supine position.
- The patient lies supine on the X-ray table, with the median sagittal plane coincident with, and at right angles to, the midline of the table and table Bucky.
- The anterior superior iliac spines should be equidistant from the table top.
- The hips and knees are flexed, and the feet are placed with their plantar aspect on the table top to reduce the lumbar arch and bring the lumbar region of the vertebral column parallel with the detector.
- The detector should be placed in the portrait position (longitudinal) to include the lower thoracic vertebrae and the sacro-iliac joints and is centred at the level of the lower costal margin.
- The exposure should be made on arrested expiration, as this will cause the diaphragm to move superiorly. The air in the lungs would otherwise cause a large difference in density and poor contrast between the upper and lower lumbar vertebrae. The aim is to cover all lumbar vertebrae with abdominal tissue.

Direction and Location of the X-ray Beam

- The collimated vertical beam is centred over the midline at the level of the lower costal margin (L3).

Essential Image Characteristics (Fig. 2.52b)

- The image should show the vertebrae from T12 down, to include all of the sacro-iliac joints.
- Rotation can be assessed by ensuring that the sacro-iliac joints are equidistant from the spine.
- The exposure and image processing should enable bony detail to be discerned throughout the region of interest.

Expected DRL: DAP 1.5 Gy·cm², ESD 5.7 mGy

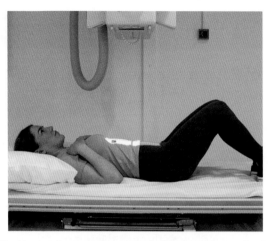

Fig. 2.52a Positioning for an antero-posterior lumbar spine projection.

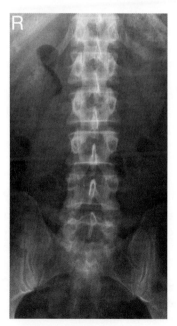

Fig. 2.52b Example of an antero-posterior lumbar spine radiograph.

LUMBAR SPINE – LATERAL

Position of Patient and Image Receptor (Fig. 2.53a)

- As with the antero-posterior projection, the lateral projection can also be obtained in the lying or erect position. The technique below describes the lying position.
- The patient lies on either side on the X-ray table utilising the Bucky. If there is any degree of scoliosis, then the most appropriate lateral position will be such that the concavity of the curve is towards the X-ray tube.
- The arms should be raised and resting on the pillow in front of the patient's head. The knees and hips are flexed for stability.
- The coronal plane running through the centre of the spine should coincide with, and be perpendicular to, the midline of the imaging detector within the table Bucky mechanism.
- Non-opaque pads may be placed under the waist and knees, as necessary, to bring the vertebral column parallel to the detector.
- The image detector is centred at the level of the lower costal margin.
- The exposure should be made on arrested expiration.
- This projection can also be undertaken erect with the patient standing or sitting, if requested, for example to demonstrate increased loss of vertebral body height or to assess stability when weight bearing.

Direction and Location of the X-ray Beam

- The collimated vertical beam is centred at right angles to the line of the spinous processes and towards a point 7.5 cm anterior to the third lumbar spinous process at the level of the lower costal margin.

Essential Image Characteristics (Fig. 2.53b)

- The image should show the vertebrae from T12 downwards, to include the lumbar sacral junction.
- Ideally, the projection will produce visualisation of the intervertebral disc space, with individual vertebral endplates superimposed.

- The cortices at the posterior and anterior margins of the vertebral body should also be superimposed.
- The imaging factors selected must produce image detail sufficient for diagnosis from T12 to L5/S1, including the spinous processes.

Expected DRL: DAP 2.5 Gy·cm², ESD 10 mGy

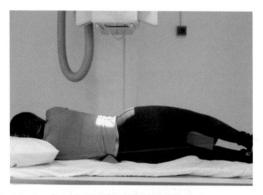

Fig. 2.53a Positioning for a lateral lumbar spine projection.

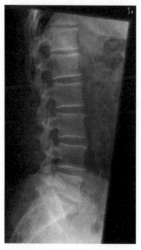

Fig. 2.53b Example of a lateral lumbar spine radiograph.

LUMBAR SPINE – OBLIQUE

Position of Patient and Image Receptor (Fig. 2.54a)

- The patient is positioned supine on the X-ray table, utilising the table Bucky detector, and is then rotated 45 degrees to the right and left sides in turn.
- The hips and knees are flexed, and the patient may be supported with a 45-degree foam pad placed under the trunk on the raised side.
- The patient's arms can be moved away from the sides or can be raised, with the hands resting on the pillow.

Direction and Location of the X-ray Beam

- The collimated vertical beam is centred towards the midclavicular line on the raised side at the level of the lower costal margin.

Essential Image Characteristics (Fig. 2.54b)

- The degree of obliquity should be such that the posterior elements of the vertebrae are aligned to show the appearance of a Scottie dog.

Notes

- These projections demonstrate the pars interarticularis and the apophyseal joints on the side nearest the image receptor. Both sides are taken for comparison.

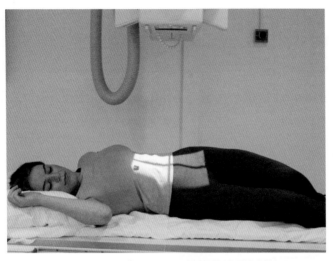

Fig. 2.54a Positioning for an oblique lumbar spine projection.

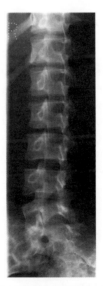

Fig. 2.54b Example of an oblique lumbar spine radiograph showing the appearance of a 'Scottie dog' sign to exclude a pars defect.

LUMBO-SACRAL JUNCTION (L5–S1) – LATERAL

Position of Patient and Image Receptor (Fig. 2.55a)

- The patient lies on either side on the X-ray table, utilising the table Bucky detector, with the arms raised and the hands resting on the pillow. The knees and hips are flexed slightly for stability.
- The dorsal aspect of the trunk should be at right angles to the image detector within the Bucky. This can be assessed by palpating the iliac crests or the posterior superior iliac spines.
- The coronal plane running through the centre of the spine should coincide with, and be perpendicular to, the midline of the image detector.
- The image detector is centred at the level of the fifth lumbar spinous process.
- Non-opaque pads may be placed under the waist and knees, as necessary, to bring the vertebral column parallel to the image detector.

Direction and Location of the X-ray Beam

- The collimated vertical beam is centred at right angles to the lumbo-sacral region and towards a point 7.5 cm anterior to the fifth lumbar spinous process. This is found at the level of the tubercle of the iliac crest or midway between the level of the upper border of the iliac crest and the anterior superior iliac spine.
- If the patient has particularly large hips and the spine is not parallel with the table top, then a 5-degree caudal angulation may be required to clear the joint space.

Essential Image Characteristics (Fig. 2.55b)

- The area of interest should include the fifth lumbar vertebra and the first sacral segment.
- A clear joint space should be demonstrated.

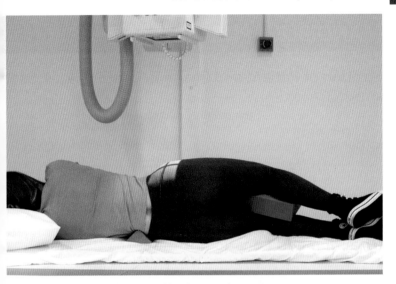

Fig. 2.55a Positioning for a lateral lumbo-sacral junction projection.

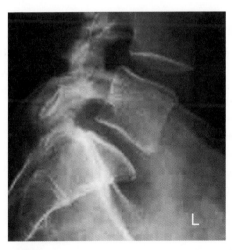

Fig. 2.55b Example of a lateral lumbo-sacral junction radiograph.

MANDIBLE – POSTERO-ANTERIOR

Position of Patient and Image Receptor (Fig. 2.56a)

- The patient sits erect facing the vertical detector/Bucky mechanism (in the case of trauma the projection may be taken anteroposteriorly).
- The patient's median sagittal plane should be coincident and perpendicular to the midline of the vertical detector and the head is then adjusted to bring the orbito-meatal baseline perpendicular to the image detector.
- The EAMs should be equidistant from the image detector.

Direction and Location of the X-ray Beam

- The collimated central ray is directed perpendicular to the image detector and centred in the midline at the levels of the angles of the mandible.

Essential Image Characteristics (Fig. 2.56b)

- The whole of the mandible from the lower portions of the temporo-mandibular joint (TMJ) to the symphysis menti must be included in the image.
- There should be no rotation evident.

Additional Considerations

- This projection demonstrates the body and rami of the mandible and may show transverse or oblique fractures not evident on other projections or using orthopantomography/dental panoramic tomography.
- The region of the symphysis menti is superimposed over the cervical vertebra but fractures in this region are often better demonstrated in this way than by orthopantomography/dental panoramic tomography.

Notes

- A 10-degree cranial angulation of the beam may be required to demonstrate the mandibular condyles and TMJs.

Expected DRL: ESD 1.24 mGy

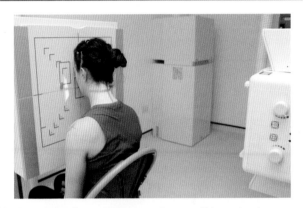

Fig. 2.56a Positioning for a postero-anterior mandible projection.

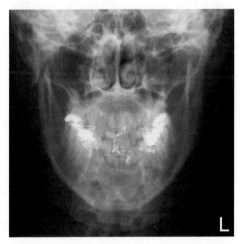

Fig. 2.56b Example of a postero-anterior mandible radiograph.

MANDIBLE – LATERAL OBLIQUE 30-DEGREE CRANIAL

Position of Patient and Image Receptor (Figs. 2.57a,b)

- The patient sits erect, or alternatively lies in the supine position with the trunk is rotated slightly to allow the side of the face being examined to come into contact with the image detector. In the supine position a thin wedge pad is used to support the head.
- The median sagittal plane should be parallel with the image detector and the interpupillary line perpendicular to both.
- The neck may be extended slightly to clear the mandible from the spine.
- The long axis of the image detector should be parallel with the long axis of the mandible and the lower border positioned 2 cm below the lower border of the mandible.

Direction and Location of the X-ray Beam

- The collimated beam is angled 30 degrees cranially and is centred 5 cm inferior to the angle of the mandible remote from the detector.
- Collimate to include the whole of the mandible and TMJ (include the EAM at the edge of the collimation field).

Essential Image Characteristics (Fig. 2.57c)

- The body and ramus of each side of the mandible should not be superimposed.
- The image should include the whole mandible from the TMJ to the symphysis menti.

Additional Considerations

- Do not mistake the mandibular canal, which transmits the inferior alveolar nerve, for a fracture.

Notes

- In cases of injury both sides should be examined to demonstrate a possible contre-coup fracture.
- If the patient is unable to move due to injury or disability, this technique can also be undertaken with the patient in a supine position, with a horizontal beam.

Expected DRL: ESD 0.66 mGy

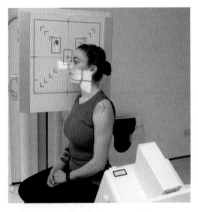

Fig. 2.57a Positioning for a lateral oblique mandible projection – erect.

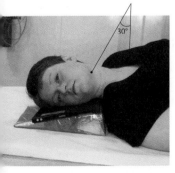

Fig. 2.57b Positioning for a lateral oblique mandible projection – supine.

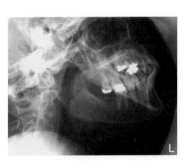

Fig. 2.57c Example of a lateral oblique mandible radiograph.

ORBITS – OCCIPITO-MENTAL (MODIFIED)

This is a frequently undertaken projection used to assess injuries to the orbital region (e.g. blow-out fracture of the orbital floor) and to exclude the presence of metallic foreign bodies in the eyes prior to magnetic resonance imaging (MRI) investigations.

Position of Patient and Image Receptor (Fig. 2.58a)

- The projection is best performed with the patient seated facing the vertical detector/Bucky.
- The patient's nose and chin are placed in contact with the midline of the vertical detector and then the head is adjusted to bring the orbito-meatal baseline to a 35-degree angle to the detector.
- The horizontal central line of the vertical detector should be at the level of the midpoint of the orbits.
- Ensure the median sagittal plane is at right angles to the image detector by checking that the outer canthi of the eyes and the EAMs are equidistant from the image detector.

Direction and Location of the X-ray Beam

- The X-ray tube should be centred to the vertical detector/ Bucky using a collimated horizontal beam before positioning is undertaken.

Essential Image Characteristics (Figs. 2.58b,c)

- The orbits should be roughly circular in appearance (they will be more oval in the occipito-mental projection).
- The petrous ridges should appear in the lower third of the maxillary sinuses. There should be no rotation.

Notes

- If the examination is purely to exclude foreign bodies in the orbit, tight 'letter box' collimation to the orbital region should be applied.

■ When using a vertical DR detector the sealed nature of the equipment should mean no additional cleaning is needed. However, if you are using a computed radiography cassette for this examination to detect foreign bodies it should be regularly cleaned to avoid small artefacts on the screens being confused with foreign bodies.

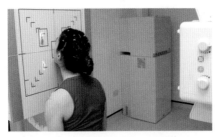

Fig. 2.58a Positioning for orbits – occipito-mental projection.

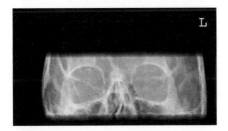

Fig. 2.58b Collimation used for a foreign-body projection

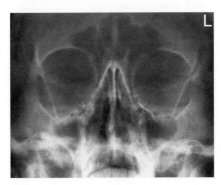

Fig. 2.58c Example of a radiograph of the orbits.

ORTHOPANTOMOGRAPHY/DENTAL PANORAMIC TOMOGRAPHY

Patient Preparation

- The patient should remove all radio-opaque objects from the head and neck areas.
- The unit should be readied in the start position and raised sufficiently to allow the patient to walk into the equipment. The examination can be carried out with the patient either standing or seated.
- Careful explanation of the procedure must be given to the patient as the exposure times vary from 12 seconds for newer equipment and up to 20 seconds for older panoramic units.
- The technique described below outlines the typical procedure for a DR orthopantomography machine.

Position of Patient and Image Receptor (Fig. 2.59a)

- The unit is placed in the start position. Position a biteblock on the machine or chin rest (dependent on the equipment).
- Ask the patient to walk straight into the machine, gripping the handles if available, and ask them to adopt the 'ski position'. The patient's head should be tilted down towards the floor so that the Frankfort plane is parallel to the floor. In this position the ala–tragus line is 5 degrees caudal.
- Turn on positioning lights and ensure the sagittal plane light is down the middle of the face. The Frankfort plane should be 5 degrees down from the ala–tragus line. The antero-posterior light should be centred distal to the upper lateral incisor (i.e. the lateral/canine interproximal space).
- Stand behind the patient and check the symmetry of the position; adjust if needed by holding the shoulders. Close the head restraints.
- Ask the patient to close their lips and press their tongue to the roof of their mouth. Closing the lips around the biteblock reduces the air shadow that can be mistaken for caries where it overlies the dentition in the premolar region.
- Explain again that the patient must stay still for about 20 seconds.
- Make the exposure (Fig. 2.59b).

Notes

■ The technique is plagued with problems relating to positioning errors and patient movement – see 13th Edition of *Clark's Positioning in Radiography* for further information and essential characteristics.

Expected DRL: ESD 9.0 mGy

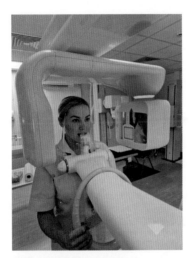

Fig. 2.59a Positioning for orthopantomography.

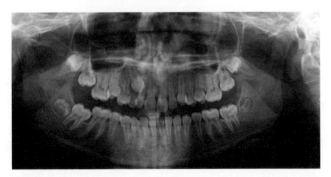

Fig. 2.59b Example of a correctly positioned orthopantomographic projection.

PELVIS – ANTERO-POSTERIOR

Position of Patient and Image Receptor (Fig. 2.60a)

- This technique can be undertaken in the supine or erect position; however, it is typically conducted in the supine position described here.
- The patient lies supine and symmetrical on the X-ray table, utilising the table Bucky, with the median sagittal plane perpendicular to the table top. The midline of the patient must coincide with the centred primary beam and table detector Bucky mechanism.
- To avoid pelvic rotation the anterior superior iliac spines must be equidistant from the table top.
- The limbs are slightly abducted and internally rotated to bring the femoral necks parallel to the image detector.
- In certain clinical circumstances, an orthopaedic templating ball bearing may be used. When placed, this ball bearing is generally positioned in the groin area, approximately level with the greater trochanter to ensure equivalent magnification of the ball bearing and the bony anatomy.

Direction and Location of the X-ray Beam

- The collimated vertical beam is centred over the midline midway between the upper border of the symphysis pubis and anterior superior iliac spines to include the whole of the pelvis and proximal femora. The upper edge of the image detector should be 5 cm above the upper border of the iliac crest.
- The centre of the image detector is placed level with the upper border of the symphysis pubis for the hips and upper femora (low-centred pelvis).

Essential Image Characteristics (Fig. 2.60b)

- For the basic pelvis projection, both iliac crests and proximal femora, including the lesser trochanters, should be visible on the image.
- The exposure should be adequate to visualise the bones of the posterior pelvis (sacrum and sacro-iliac joints) and the proximal femora.

Notes

■ Internal rotation of the limb compensates for the X-ray beam divergence when centring in the midline. The resultant image will show both greater and lesser trochanters.

Expected DRL: DAP 2.2 Gy·cm², ESD 4 mGy

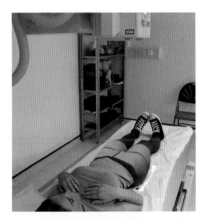

Fig. 2.60a Positioning for an antero-posterior pelvic projection.

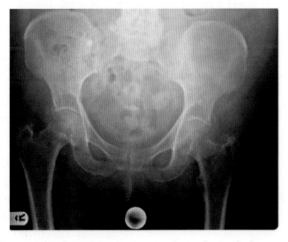

Fig. 2.60b Example of an antero-posterior pelvis radiograph showing use of an orthopaedic templating ball bearing.

189

SACRO-ILIAC JOINTS – POSTERO-ANTERIOR

The sacrum is situated posteriorly between the two iliac bones, the adjacent surfaces forming the sacro-iliac joints. These joint surfaces are oblique in direction, sloping backward, inward and downward.

In the prone position the oblique divergent rays coincide with the direction of the joints.

Position of Patient and Image Receptor (Figs. 2.61a,b)

- The patient lies prone on the X-ray table with the median sagittal perpendicular to the table top and table Bucky detector.
- The posterior superior iliac spines should be equidistant from the table top to avoid rotation.
- The midline of the patient should coincide with the centred primary beam and table Bucky mechanism.
- The image detector is positioned so that the central ray passes though the centre of the detector.

Direction and Location of the X-ray Beam

- The collimated vertical beam is centred in the midline at the level of the posterior superior iliac spines.
- The central ray is angled 5–15 degrees caudally from the vertical depending on the angulation of the patient's sacrum, which is generally greater in females due to the natural increased L5/S1 lordosis.
- The primary beam is collimated to the area of interest.

Notes

- The postero-anterior projection demonstrates the joints more effectively than the antero-posterior projection. It also reduces the radiation dose to the gonads compared with the antero-posterior projection.
- Additional imaging may be required as some pathologies, such as sacro-iliitis, require more detailed demonstration of the joints with the aid of CT/MRI.

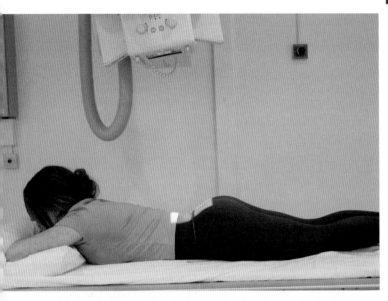

Fig. 2.61a Positioning for a postero-anterior sacro-iliac joint projection.

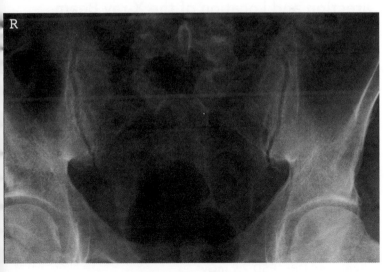

Fig. 2.61b Example of a normal postero-anterior sacro-iliac joints radiograph.

SACRUM – ANTERO-POSTERIOR

The antero-posterior projection demonstrates both sacro-iliac joints and the sacrum on one image and can be done when the patient is unable to lie prone.

The technique utilises the table Bucky mechanism and image detector.

Position of Patient and Image Receptor (Fig. 2.62a)

- The patient lies supine and symmetrical on the X-ray table with the median sagittal plane perpendicular to the table top.
- The image detector is positioned so that the central ray passes through the midline of the patient.
- To avoid rotation the anterior superior iliac spines must be equidistant from the table top.
- The shoulders are raised over a pillow and the knees may be flexed over foam pads for comfort and to reduce pelvic tilt.

Direction and Location of the X-ray Beam

- The collimated vertical beam is centred in the midline at a level midway between the anterior superior iliac spines and superior border of the symphysis pubis.
- The central ray is directed 5–15 degrees cranially depending on the sex of the patient due to the natural angulation of the male/female pelvis and lordosis of the lower lumbar spine.

Notes (Fig. 2.62b)

- The sacrum may be required to be visualised in detail to assess the sacral foramina and body when a fracture is suspected. Also, although the sacro-iliac joints are best demonstrated in the postero-anterior projection this may not be a feasible position for the patient and the antero-posterior sacrum technique may be used as an alternative.

Expected DRL: ESD 2.9 mGy*

*Based on a small sample size.

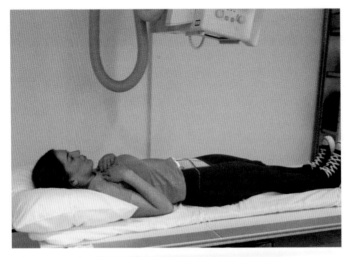

Fig. 2.62a Positioning for an antero-posterior sacrum projection.

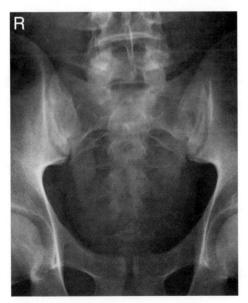

Fig. 2.62b Example of an antero-posterior sacrum radiograph.

SACRUM – LATERAL

This is a non-routine examination that delivers a large radiation dose to the patient. CT is the alternative imaging technique that can be used to identify discrete fractures, particularly in the older patient.

Position of Patient and Image Receptor (Fig. 2.63a)

- The patient lies on either side on the X-ray table, utilising the table Bucky mechanism, with the arms raised and the hands resting on the pillow. The knees and hips are flexed slightly for stability.
- The dorsal aspect of the trunk should be at right angles to the image detector. This can be assessed by palpating the iliac crests or the posterior superior iliac spines. The coronal plane running through the centre of the spine should coincide with, and be perpendicular to, the midline of the table detector.
- The image detector and Bucky mechanism is centred to coincide with the central ray at the level of the midpoint of the sacrum.

Direction and Location of the X-ray Beam

- The collimated vertical X-ray beam is directed towards the long axis of the sacrum. It is centred midway between the posterior superior iliac spines and the sacro-coccygeal junction.

Essential Image Characteristics (Fig. 2.63b)

- The image should include all of the sacrum from the lumbar sacral junction down to the sacro-coccygeal junction.
- The posterior collimation and imaging exposure factors should be sufficient to allow demonstration of the posterior spinous tubercle.

Additional Considerations

- Fractures may be missed if the image is underexposed or if the pelvis is rotated.

Notes

■ If using an AEC, inadequate centring (usually posteriorly) will result in an underexposed image.

Expected DRL: ESD 8.12 mGy*

*Based on a small sample size.

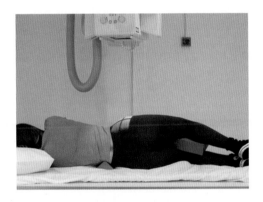

Fig. 2.63a Positioning for a lateral sacrum projection.

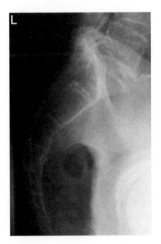

Fig. 2.63b Example of a lateral sacrum radiograph.

SCAPHOID – POSTERO-ANTERIOR WITH ULNAR DEVIATION

For suspected scaphoid fractures, three or more projections may be taken (dependent on local protocol). These normally include the postero-anterior and lateral wrist projections (see Wrist – Postero-anterior and Wrist – Lateral), plus one or more of the four scaphoid projections described in this book.

Position of Patient and Image Receptor (Fig. 2.64a)

- The patient is seated alongside the table, with the affected side nearest to the table.
- The arm is extended across the table with the elbow flexed and the forearm pronated.
- If possible, the shoulder, elbow and wrist should be at the level of the table top.
- The wrist is positioned over the centre of the image detector and the hand is adducted (ulnar deviation).
- Ensure that the radial and ulnar styloid processes are equidistant from the image detector.
- The hand and lower forearm may be immobilised using sandbags.

Direction and Location of the X-ray Beam

- The collimated vertical beam is centred to the scaphoid.

Essential Image Characteristics (Fig. 2.64b)

- The image should include the distal end of the radius and ulna and the proximal end of the metacarpals.
- The joint space around the scaphoid should be demonstrated clearly.

Notes

- When the image is undertaken specifically for a scaphoid projection, the wrist should be in ulnar deviation.

Expected DRL: ESD 0.072 mGy

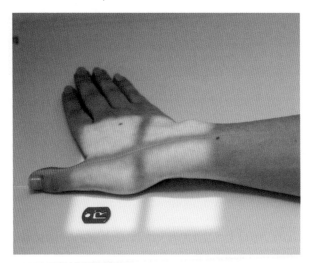

Fig. 2.64a Positioning for a postero-anterior projection of the scaphoid with ulnar deviation.

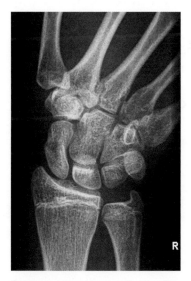

Fig. 2.64b Example of a postero-anterior scaphoid radiograph with ulnar deviation.

SCAPHOID – ANTERIOR OBLIQUE WITH ULNAR DEVIATION

Position of Patient and Image Receptor (Fig. 2.65a)

- From the postero-anterior position, the hand and wrist are rotated 45 degrees externally and placed centrally over the image detector. The hand should remain adducted in ulnar deviation.
- The hand may be supported in position, with a non-opaque pad placed under the thumb.
- The forearm may be immobilised using a sandbag.

Direction and Location of the X-ray Beam

- The collimated vertical beam is centred to the scaphoid.

Essential Image Characteristics (Fig. 2.65b)

- The image should include the distal end of the radius and ulna and the proximal end of the metacarpals.
- The scaphoid should be seen clearly, with its long axis parallel to the image detector.

Additional Considerations

- A carpal fracture is a break of one of the eight small bones of the carpus. These bones are the scaphoid, lunate, capitate, triquetrum, hamate, pisiform, trapezium and trapezoid. The scaphoid is, however, the most commonly fractured.

> **Expected DRL: ESD 0.072 mGy**

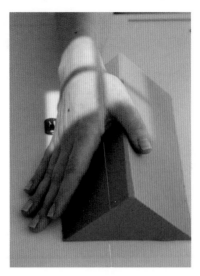

Fig. 2.65a Positioning for a scaphoid anterior oblique projection with ulnar deviation.

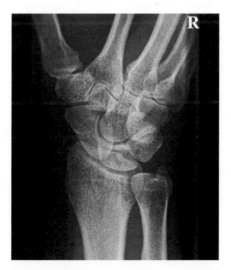

Fig. 2.65b Example of a scaphoid anterior oblique radiograph with ulnar deviation.

SCAPHOID – POSTERIOR OBLIQUE

Position of Patient and Image Receptor (Fig. 2.66a)

- From the anterior oblique position, the hand and wrist are rotated externally through 90 degrees, such that the posterior aspect of the hand and wrist are at 45 degrees to the image detector.
- The wrist may then be supported on a 45-degree non-opaque foam pad.
- The forearm may be immobilised using a sandbag if required.

Direction and Location of the X-ray Beam

- The collimated vertical beam is centred over the scaphoid.

Essential Image Characteristics (Fig. 2.66b)

- The image should include the distal end of the radius and ulna and the proximal end of the metacarpals.
- The pisiform should be seen clearly in profile situated anterior to the triquetral.
- The long axis of the scaphoid should be seen perpendicular to the image detector.

Expected DRL: ESD 0.072 mGy

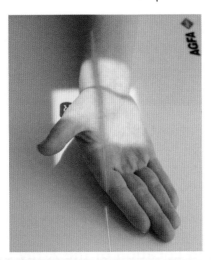

Fig. 2.66a Positioning for a posterior oblique scaphoid projection.

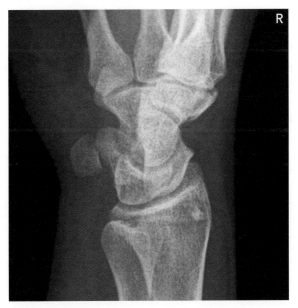

Fig. 2.66b Example of a posterior oblique scaphoid radiograph.

SCAPHOID – POSTERO-ANTERIOR WITH ULNAR DEVIATION AND 30-DEGREE CRANIAL ANGLE

Position of Patient and Image Receptor (Fig. 2.67a)

- The patient and image detector are positioned as for the postero-anterior scaphoid with ulnar deviation.
- The wrist must be positioned to allow the X-ray tube to be angled at 30 degrees along the long axis of the scaphoid.

Direction and Location of the X-ray Beam

- The collimated vertical beam is angled 30 degrees cranially and centred to the scaphoid.

Essential Image Characteristics (Fig. 2.67b)

- This projection elongates the scaphoid, and with ulnar deviation it demonstrates the space surrounding the scaphoid.

Additional Considerations

- Fracture of the waist of the scaphoid may not be clearly visible, if at all, at presentation. It carries a high risk of delayed avascular necrosis of the distal pole, which can cause severe disability.
- If suspected clinically, the patient may be re-examined after 10 days of immobilisation; otherwise, MRI may offer immediate diagnosis.

> **Expected DRL: ESD 0.072 mGy**

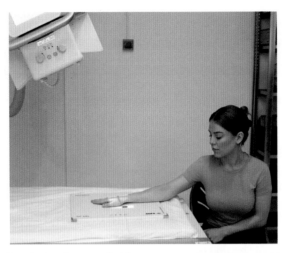

Fig. 2.67a Positioning for a scaphoid postero-anterior projection with ulnar deviation and 30-degree cranial angle.

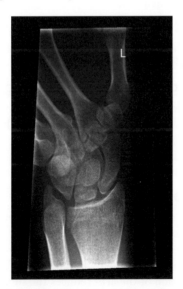

Fig. 2.67b Example of a scaphoid postero-anterior radiograph with ulnar deviation and 30-degree cranial angle.

SHOULDER GIRDLE – ANTERO-POSTERIOR (15-DEGREE) ERECT

Position of Patient and Image Receptor (Fig. 2.68a)

- The patient stands with the affected shoulder against the image detector and the torso is rotated approximately 15 degrees towards the affected side to bring the plane of the glenoid fossa perpendicular to the image detector.
- The arm is supinated and slightly abducted away from the body.
- The image detector is positioned so that its upper border is at least 5 cm above the shoulder to ensure that the oblique rays do not project the shoulder off the edge of the final image.
- The patient should be asked to rotate their head away from the side under examination to avoid superimposition of the chin over the medial end of the clavicle.

Direction and Location of the X-ray Beam

- The collimated horizontal beam is directed to the palpable coracoid process of the scapula.

Essential Image Characteristics (Fig. 2.68b)

- The image should demonstrate the head and proximal end of the humerus, the inferior angle of the scapula and the whole of the clavicle including the sterno-clavicular joint.
- The head of the humerus should be seen *slightly* overlapping the glenoid cavity but separate from the acromion process.

Additional Considerations

- This is a general survey image of the shoulder which demonstrates most of the anatomy to an acceptable standard. For focused imaging of glenohumeral joint, such as for impingement or calcified tendonitis, see the alternative techniques described.
- Too much abduction of the arm reduces the subacromial space, making it difficult to diagnose pathology in this area.

Expected DRL: ESD 0.5 mGy

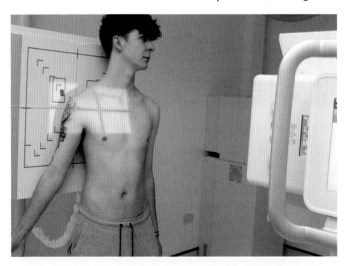

Fig. 2.68a Positioning for an antero-posterior shoulder girdle projection.

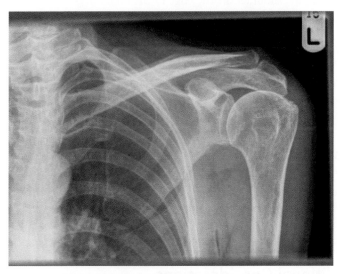

Fig. 2.68b Example of an antero-posterior shoulder girdle radiograph.

SHOULDER GIRDLE – ANTERO-POSTERIOR (GLENOHUMERAL JOINT) – MODIFIED (GRASHEY PROJECTION)

Position of Patient and Image Receptor (Fig. 2.69a)

- The patient stands with the affected shoulder against the image detector and the torso is rotated approximately 35–45 degrees towards the affected side to bring the plane of the glenoid fossa perpendicular to the image detector.
- The arm is supinated and slightly abducted away from the body.
- The image detector is positioned so that its upper border is at least 5 cm above the shoulder to ensure that the oblique rays do not project the shoulder off the edge of the final image.
- The patient should be asked to rotate their head away from the side under examination to avoid superimposition of the chin over the medial end of the clavicle.

Direction and Location of the X-ray Beam

- The collimated horizontal beam is directed to the palpable coracoid process of the scapula.

Essential Image Characteristics (Fig. 2.69b)

- The image should demonstrate a clear joint space between the head of the humerus and the glenoid cavity.
- The image should demonstrate the head and the greater and lesser tuberosities of the humerus, together with the lateral aspect of the scapula and the distal end of the clavicle.

Additional Considerations

- This projection is useful for demonstrating the glenohumeral joint in joint instability and for narrowing seen in arthritis.

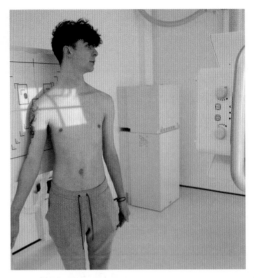

Fig. 2.69a Positioning for a shoulder girdle – antero-posterior modified (Grashey) projection.

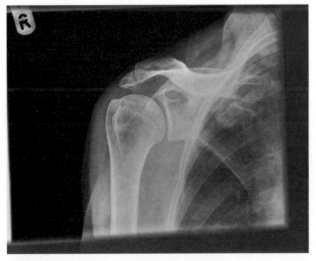

Fig. 2.69b Example of a Grashey projection radiograph.

SHOULDER – SUPERO-INFERIOR (AXIAL)

Position of Patient and Image Receptor (Fig. 2.70a)

- The patient is seated with the affected side adjacent to the table, which is lowered to waist level.
- The image detector is placed on the table top, and the arm under examination is abducted over the table.
- The patient leans towards the table to reduce the ORD and to ensure that the glenoid cavity is included in the image.
- The elbow can remain flexed, but the arm should be abducted to a minimum of 45 degrees, injury permitting. If only limited abduction is possible, the receptor may be supported on pads to reduce the ORD.

Direction and Location of the X-ray Beam

- The collimated vertical beam is centred over the mid-glenohumeral joint. X-ray tube angulation of 8 degrees towards the elbow may be necessary to coincide with the plane of the glenoid cavity.
- If there is a large ORD it may be necessary to increase the overall FRD to reduce magnification.

Essential Image Characteristics (Fig. 2.70b)

- The image must demonstrate the head of the humerus, the acromion process, the coracoid process and the glenoid cavity of the scapula.

Additional Considerations

- Trauma patients will have severe difficulty in abducting their arm and should not be forced to do so. In such cases it is recommended that the apical oblique projection is undertaken (as described in the 13th Edition of *Clark's Positioning in Radiography*). However, if that is not possible then an anterior oblique ('Y') projection can be undertaken.

Expected DRL: ESD 0.58 mGy

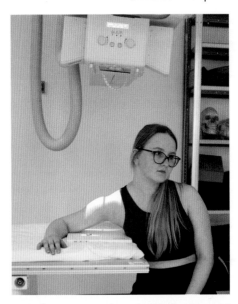

Fig. 2.70a Positioning for a supero-inferior (axial) shoulder projection,

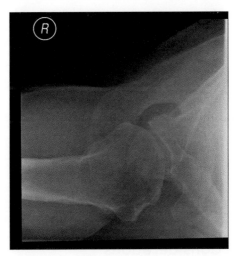

Fig. 2.70b Example of a supero-inferior (axial) shoulder radiograph.

SHOULDER – ANTERIOR OBLIQUE ('Y' PROJECTION)

Position of Patient and Image Receptor (Figs. 2.71a,b)

- The patient stands or sits facing the vertical image detector/Bucky with the lateral aspect of the injured arm against the image detector. The shoulder is adjusted so that the axilla is in the centre of the image detector.
- The unaffected shoulder is rotated to make the angle between the trunk and the detector approximately 60 degrees. A line joining the medial and lateral borders of the scapula is now at right angles to the image detector.
- The image detector is positioned to include the superior and inferior borders of the scapula.

Direction and Location of the X-ray Beam

- The collimated horizontal beam is centred towards the medial border of the scapula and centred to the head of the humerus.
- Collimate to include the region 2 cm above the palpable acromion process superiorly, just below the inferior aspect of the scapula inferiorly, the posterior skin margin and 2 cm of the rib cage anteriorly.

Essential Image Characteristics (Fig. 2.71c)

- The body of the scapula should be at right angles to the image detector, and thus demonstrate the scapula and the proximal end of the humerus clear of the rib cage.
- The exposure should demonstrate the position of the head of the humerus in relation to the glenoid cavity between the coracoid and acromion processes.

Additional Considerations

- The 'Y' projection is generally undertaken as a result of scapula trauma or to see multi-part proximal humeral fracture fragments.

- If the arm is immobilised and no abduction of the arm is possible, then an anterior oblique projection may be taken as an alternative to an axial projection.
- Over- or under-rotation of the torso will result in superimposition of the rib cage over the region of interest.

Expected DRL: ESD 0.73 mGy

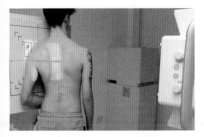 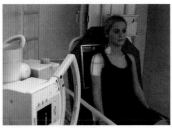

Figs. 2.71a,b Positioning for an anterior oblique shoulder projection in the erect position and an alternative 'reverse' position for use on a trolley.

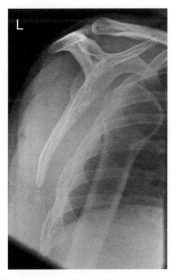

Fig. 2.71c Example of an anterior oblique 'Y' projection radiograph showing an anterior dislocation of the humeral head from the glenoid fossa.

SINUSES – OCCIPITO-MENTAL

This projection is designed to project the petrous part of the temporal bone below the floor of the maxillary sinuses so that fluid levels or pathological changes in the lower part of the sinuses can be clearly visualised.

Position of Patient and Image Receptor (Fig. 2.72a)

- The projection is best performed with the patient seated facing the vertical detector/Bucky.
- The patient's nose and chin are placed in contact with the midline of the detector and then the head is adjusted to bring the orbito-meatal baseline at a 45-degree angle to the detector.
- The horizontal central line of the Bucky/detector should be at the level of the lower orbital margins.
- The median sagittal plane is at right angles to the Bucky/detector by ensuring the outer canthi of the eyes and the EAMs are equidistant.
- The patient should open their mouth as wide as possible prior to exposure. This will allow the posterior part of the sphenoid sinuses to be projected through the mouth.

Direction and Location of the X-ray Beam

- The collimated horizontal beam should be centred to the Bucky/detector before positioning is undertaken.
- To check the beam is centred properly, the crosslines on the Bucky/detector should coincide with the patient's anterior nasal spine.
- Collimate to include all of the sinuses.

Essential Image Characteristics (Fig. 2.72b)

- The petrous ridges must appear below the floors of the maxillary sinuses.
- There should be no rotation.

Notes

- Always check the baseline angle immediately before exposure as this is an uncomfortable position to maintain.

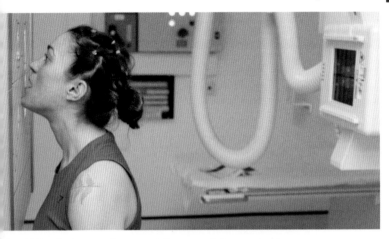

Fig. 2.72a Positioning for an occipito-mental sinus projection.

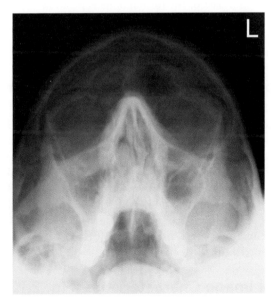

Fig. 2.72b Example of an occipito-mental sinus projection, showing a polyp in the right maxillary sinus.

SKULL – OCCIPITO-FRONTAL

Occipito-frontal projections can be undertaken with the patient erect or (less commonly) prone on the X-ray table with different degrees of beam angulation.

Position of Patient and Image Receptor (Figs. 2.73a,b)

- The patient is seated facing the erect Bucky/detector so that the median sagittal plane is coincident with the midline of the image detector and is also perpendicular to it.
- The neck is flexed so that the orbito-meatal baseline is perpendicular to the image detector. This can usually be achieved by ensuring the nose and forehead are in contact with the Bucky/detector. Ensure the mid part of the frontal bone is positioned in the centre of the Bucky/detector.
- The patient may place the palms of each hand either side of the head (out of the primary beam) for stability.

Direction and Location of the X-ray Beam

- The collimated horizontal beam is directed perpendicular to the Bucky/detector along the median sagittal plane or angled caudally 10, 15 or 20 degrees, dependent on the department protocol and anatomical area.
- To ensure the beam is centred properly the crosslines on the Bucky/detector should coincide with the patient's glabella.
- The beam collimation should include the vertex of the skull superiorly, the region immediately below the base of the occipital bone inferiorly and the lateral skin margins. It is important to ensure the tube is centred to the Bucky detector.

Essential Image Characteristics (Fig. 2.73c)

- All the cranial bones should be included in the image, including the skin margins. It is important to ensure the skull is not rotated.

Additional Considerations

■ This examination may be undertaken with 10-, 15- or 20-degree caudal beam angulations. This will result in the petrous ridges appearing more inferiorly in the orbit.

Notes

■ Patients often find it difficult to maintain or achieve their orbi-to-meatal baseline perpendicular to the image receptor as it is an uncomfortable position. Modifications in tube angulation may accommodate this.

Expected DRL: ESD 1.8 mGy

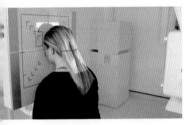

Fig. 2.73a Positioning for an occipito-frontal skull projection.

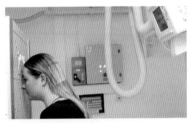

Fig. 2.73b Positioning for an occipito-frontal 20-degree caudal skull projection.

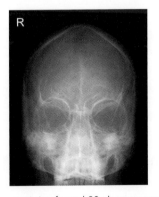

Fig. 2.73c Example of an occipito-frontal 20-degree caudal angulation skull projection.

SKULL – OCCIPITO-FRONTAL 30-DEGREE CRANIAL (REVERSE TOWNE'S)

Position of Patient and Image Receptor (Fig. 2.74a)

- This projection is usually undertaken with the patient in the erect position facing the erect Bucky/image detector, although it may be performed with the patient prone, on the X-ray table.
- Initially the patient is asked to place their nose and forehead against the image detector. The head is adjusted to bring the median sagittal plane at right angles to the image detector, so it is coincident with its midline.
- The orbito-meatal baseline should be perpendicular to the image detector.
- The patient may place their hands on the Bucky/detector for stability.

Direction and Location of the X-ray Beam

- The central ray is angled cranially so it makes an angle of 30 degrees to the orbito-meatal line. Adjust the collimation field such the whole of the whole of the occipital bone and the parietal bones up to the vertex are included within the field. Avoid including the orbits in the primary beam.

Essential Image Characteristics (Fig. 2.74b)

- The sella turcica of the sphenoid bone is projected within the foramen magnum.
- The image must include all of the occipital bone and the posterior parts of the parietal bone, and the lambdoid suture should be clearly visualised.
- The skull should not be rotated.

Additional Considerations

- The foramen magnum should be clearly visualised on this projection. The margins may be obscured by incorrect angulation, thus hiding important fractures.

▪ The zygoma may be well seen on this projection and if fractured gives a clue to the presence of associated facial injury.

Notes

▪ This projection will carry a lower radiation dose to sensitive structures than the equivalent fronto-occipital 30-degree caudal projection.

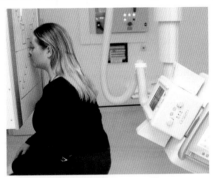

Fig. 2.74a Positioning for a reverse Towne's projection.

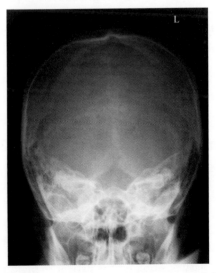

Fig. 2.74b Example of an occipito-frontal 30 degrees cranial skull radiograph.

This position may be used for a cooperative patient.

Position of Patient and Image Receptor (Figs. 2.75a,b)

- The patient sits facing the erect Bucky/detector and the head is then rotated such that the median sagittal plane is parallel to the Bucky/detector and the interpupillary line is perpendicular to the Bucky/detector.
- The shoulders may be rotated slightly to allow the correct position to be attained and the patient may grip the Bucky inferiorly for stability.
- A radiolucent pad may be placed under the chin/lower half of the face, for support.
- If using a computed radiography cassette, position the image detector such that its upper border is 5 cm above the vertex of the skull.

Direction and Location of the X-ray Beam

- The X-ray tube should be centred to the Bucky/image detector and the tracking facility utilised if available.
- Centre with a collimated horizontal beam midway between the glabella and the external occipital protuberance to a point approximately 5 cm superior and posterior to the EAM.

Essential Image Characteristics (Fig. 2.75c)

- The lateral floors of the cranial fossa should be superimposed by ensuring the interorbital line is perpendicular to the image detector and the median sagittal plane is perpendicular to the image detector.

Additional Considerations

- This is not an easy position for the patient to maintain. Check the position of all planes immediately prior to the exposure; the patient may have moved.

Notes

- This projection can also be performed with the patient prone on a floating-top table with a collimated vertical beam.

Expected DRL: ESD 1.1 mGy

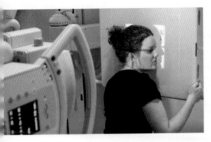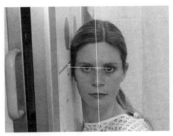

Figs. 2.75a,b Positioning for a lateral skull projection.

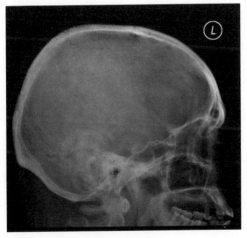

Fig. 2.75c Example of a lateral skull radiograph.

SKULL – FRONTO-OCCIPITAL (SUPINE/ TROLLEY)

Fronto-occipital projections of the skull will demonstrate the same anatomy as occipito-frontal projections. The orbits and frontal bone will be magnified as they are positioned further from the image detector.

Such projections should only be undertaken when the patient cannot be moved and must be imaged supine. These projections result in an increased radiation dose to the orbits and some loss of resolution of the anterior skull structures due to increased ORD.

Position of Patient and Image Receptor (Figs. 2.76a,b)

- The patient lies supine on the trolley (or X-ray table) with the posterior aspect of the skull resting on the gridded image detector.
- The head is adjusted to bring the median sagittal plane at right angles to the image detector and coincident with its midline. In this position the EAMs are equidistant from the image detector to ensure no rotation.
- The orbito-meatal baseline should be perpendicular to the image detector.

Direction and Location of the X-ray Beam

- All angulations for fronto-occipital projections are made cranially.
- The collimated vertical X-ray beam is directed perpendicular to the image detector along the median sagittal plane and centred to the glabella.
- The collimated field should be set to include the vertex of the skull superiorly, the base of the occipital bone inferiorly and the lateral skin margins.

Essential Image Characteristics and Notes (Fig. 2.76c)

- These are the same as for occipito-frontal projections (see Skull – Occipito-frontal and Skull).

Additional Considerations

This examination may be undertaken with 10- or 20-degree cranial beam angulations, which will result in the petrous ridges appearing more inferiorly in the orbit. For a fronto-occipital 20-degree projection when the patient can only maintain the orbito-meatal base line at 10 degrees back from the perpendicular (i.e. chin raised slightly) a 10-degree cranial angulation is applied to the tube to achieve an overall 20-degree angle.

Expected DRL: ESD 1.8 mGy

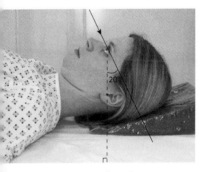

Fig. 2.76a Positioning for a fronto-occipital 20-degree cranial skull projection.

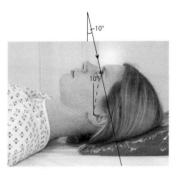

Fig. 2.76b A fronto-occipital 20-degree cranial skull projection achieved with a 10-degree tube angulation and the orbito-meatal base line raised by 10 degrees.

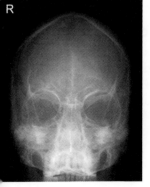

Fig. 2.76c Example of a fronto-occipital 20-degree cranial skull radiograph skull radiograph.

221

SKULL – FRONTO-OCCIPITAL 30-DEGREE CAUDAL (TOWNE'S PROJECTION) (SUPINE/TROLLEY)

Position of Patient and Image Receptor (Fig. 2.77a)

- The patient lies supine on a trolley (or X-ray table) with the posterior aspect of the skull resting on a gridded image detector.
- The head is adjusted to bring the median sagittal plane at right angles to the image detector and so that it is coincident with its midline.
- The orbito-meatal baseline should be perpendicular to the image detector.

Direction and Location of the X-ray Beam

- The collimated vertical beam is angled caudally so it makes an angle of 30 degrees to the orbito-meatal plane.
- To avoid irradiating the eyes the collimation is set to ensure the lower border coincides with the superior orbital margin and the upper border includes the skull vertex. Laterally the skin margins should also be included within the field. The top of the detector should be positioned adjacent to the vertex of the skull to ensure the beam angulation does not project the area of interest off the bottom of the image.

Essential Image Characteristics (Fig. 2.77b)

- The sella turcica of the sphenoid bone is projected to appear within the foramen magnum. The image must include all the occipital bone and the posterior parts of the parietal bone and the lambdoidal suture should be clearly visualised. The skull should not be rotated.

Additional Considerations

- The foramen magnum should be clearly seen on this projection. The margins may be obscured by incorrect angulation, thus hiding serious fractures.

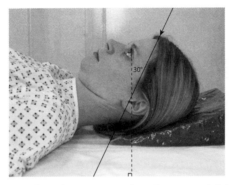

Fig. 2.77a Positioning for a fronto-occipital 30-degree caudal skull projection.

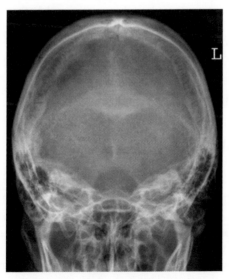

Fig. 2.77b Example of a fronto-occipital 30-degree caudal skull radiograph.

SKULL – LATERAL (SUPINE/TROLLEY)

Position of Patient and Image Receptor (Fig. 2.78a)

- The patient lies supine with the head raised and immobilised on a non-opaque skull pad. This will ensure the occipital region is included on the image.
- The head is adjusted such that the median sagittal plane is perpendicular to the table/trolley and the interpupillary line is perpendicular to the image detector.
- The gridded detector is supported vertically against the lateral aspect of the head (region of interest) parallel to the median sagittal plane with its edge at least 5 cm above the vertex of the skull.

Direction and Location of the X-ray Beam

- The collimated horizontal beam is directed parallel to the interpupillary line such that it is at right angles to the median sagittal plane.
- The centring point is midway between the glabella and the external occipital protuberance to a point approximately 5 cm superior and posterior to the EAM.
- The long axis of the detector should coincide with the long axis of the skull.

Essential Image Characteristics (Fig. 2.78b)

- As for Skull – Lateral Erect.

Additional Considerations

- Skull modality imaging is used to identify brain injury that cannot be assessed by skull radiography, so the prime modality currently used is a CT scan.
- The choice of which side to image will depend on the site of the suspected pathology. The side with the suspected pathology should be adjacent to the image detector. This will ensure the pathology is shown at the maximum resolution possible due to the minimisation of geometric sharpness. This is the projection of choice for the majority of trauma cases on a trolley if CT is not undertaken.

Expected DRL: ESD 1.1 mGy

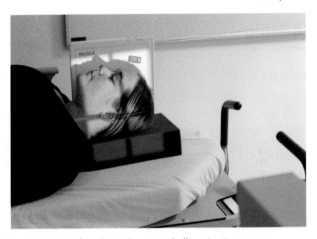

Fig. 2.78a Positioning for a lateral supine skull projection.

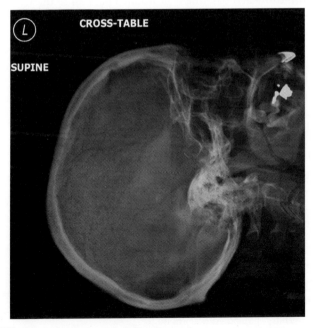

Fig. 2.78b Example of a lateral skull radiograph.

SKULL 'HEAD' – CT

Indications

- CT is used in cases of acute head trauma, suspected intracranial bleed, stroke, tumour, metastases, shunt malfunctions and when MRI is contraindicated dependent on local protocols.

Positioning of Patient and Imaging Modality (Fig. 2.79a)

- The patient is supine on the scanner table with the head resting in the head support, with arms by the patient's side. Positioning is aided by the axial, coronal and sagittal laser lights to ensure that the patient is positioned in the central axis of the scanner.
- The orbito-meatal baseline is positioned parallel to the transverse alignment. The median sagittal plane is perpendicular to the table and coincident with the sagittal alignment light.
- To ensure that the skull is symmetrically positioned, the EAMs must be equidistant from the head support and the interpupillary line is parallel to the scan plane. The head is secured by Velcro straps.
- To commence the initial 'localiser' scan the patient is moved into the gantry of the scanner until the scan reference point is at the level of the symphysis menti.

Imaging Procedure (Table 2.1)

- A lateral 'localiser' image with or without a postero-anterior image is obtained. The CT scan range should start 5 cm below and end 12 cm above the radiographic base line, i.e. from the base to the vertex of the skull.

Table 2.1 Typical protocol for 64-slice scanner – Local protocols may differ.

Scan range	Base of skull to vertex
Slice thickness	0.5–1.25 mm
Interval	0.3–1.0 mm
Algorithm/filter	Standard/brain/bone
Multiplanar reformats	2 mm axial, sagittal and coronal brain reformats 2 mm axial, sagittal and coronal bone reformats

Contrast (if indicated)	50 mL by hand or injection pump; usually 350 mg/iodine strength Same examination protocol is acquired 5 minutes post injection

Image Analysis (Figs. 2.79b,c)

■ The images are reviewed for space-occupying lesions, haemorrhage or hydrocephalus, normal basal ganglia and posterior fossa structures, major vessel vascular territory infarct, intra- or extra-axonal collections, patency of basal cisterns and foramen magnum, status of air cells of the petrous temporal bone and the presence of any fractures.

Radiation Protection/Dose

Dose reduction techniques include AEC (mA) and iterative slice reconstruction. To reduce or avoid ocular lens exposure the patient's chin is tucked down and if scanners permit the gantry may also be angled.

> **National DRL: 970 mGy.cm**

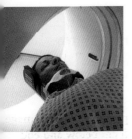

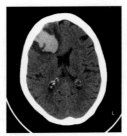

Fig. 2.79c Axial CT image demonstrating intra-cerebral haemorrhage in the right frontal lobe with surrounding oedema causing slight mass effect.

Fig. 2.79a Patient positioning for a CT head scan.

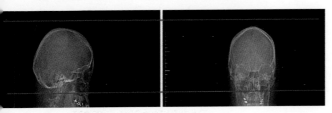

Fig. 2.79b Slice positioning for a helical CT head scan.

227

STERNUM – LATERAL

Position of Patient and Image Receptor (Fig. 2.80a)

- A vertical Bucky direct digital radiography (DDR) system is employed.
- The patient sits or stands, with either shoulder against the vertical detector.
- The median sagittal plane of the trunk is adjusted parallel to the image detector.
- The sternum is centred to the image detector.
- The patient's hands are clasped behind the back and immediately before exposure the shoulders are pulled well back.
- The image detector is centred at a level 2.5 cm below the sternal angle.
- If the patient is standing, the feet should be separated to aid stability.
- An FRD of 120–150 cm is selected to reduce magnification.

Direction and Location of the X-ray Beam

- The collimated horizontal beam is centred towards a point 2.5 cm below the sternal angle and should include the manubrium, body and xiphoid process of the sternum.
- Exposure is made on arrested full inspiration.

Essential Image Characteristics (Fig. 2.80b)

- This can be a difficult examination to interpret, especially in elderly patients, who often have heavily calcified costal cartilages.
- The image should demonstrate the full extent of the sternum, including the manubrium, body and xiphoid process.
- The contrast and density should be optimised to demonstrate the cortical margins of the sternum.

Additional Considerations

- This projection is usually taken in conjunction with a chest radiograph to search for a pneumothorax in trauma cases. Remember that the initial interpretation is often done in the emergency department by inexperienced observers; therefore, care should be exercised to ensure that the sternum is projected in the true lateral position as this is important to allow for accurate interpretation.

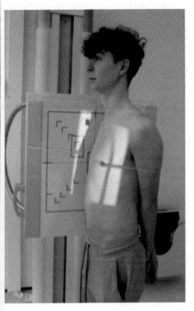

Fig. 2.80a Positioning for a lateral sternum projection.

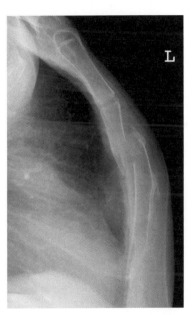

Fig. 2.80b Lateral radiograph of the sternum showing a fracture of the body with overlap of bone ends.

THORACIC SPINE
– ANTERO-POSTERIOR

Position of Patient and Image Receptor (Fig. 2.81a)

- The patient is positioned supine on the X-ray table, with the median sagittal plane perpendicular to the table top and coincident with the midline of the Bucky. This projection can also be taken in the standing/erect position against the vertical detector.
- The upper edge of the image detector should be at a level just below the prominence of the thyroid cartilage to ensure that the upper thoracic vertebrae are included.
- Exposure is made on arrested inspiration. This will cause the diaphragm to move down over the upper lumbar vertebra, thus reducing the chance of a large difference in density appearing on the image from superimposition of the lungs.

Direction and Location of the X-ray Beam

- Direct the vertical central ray at right angles to the image detector and towards a point 2.5 cm below the sternal angle.
- The beam is collimated tightly to the spine.

Essential Image Characteristics (Fig. 2.81b)

- The image should include the vertebrae from C7 to L1.
- The imaging factors should be sufficient to demonstrate bony detail for the upper as well as the thoracic lower vertebrae.

Additional Considerations

- The image detector and beam are often centred too low, thereby excluding the upper thoracic vertebrae from the image.
- The lower vertebrae are also often not included. L1 can be identified easily by the fact that it usually will not have a rib attached to it.

Expected DRL: DAP 1.0 Gy·cm², ESD 3.5 mGy

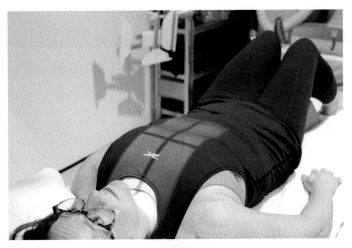

Fig. 2.81a Positioning for an antero-posterior thoracic spine projection.

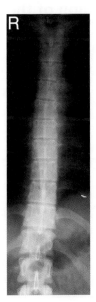

Fig. 2.81b Example of a normal antero-posterior thoracic spine radiograph.

THORACIC SPINE – LATERAL

Position of Patient and Image Receptor (Fig. 2.82a)

- The examination is usually undertaken with the patient in the lateral decubitus position on the X-ray table, although this projection can also be performed erect.
- The median sagittal plane should be parallel to the image detector and the midline of the axilla coincident with the midline of the Bucky/detector.
- The arms should be raised well above the head.
- The head can be supported with a pillow, and pads may be placed between the knees for the patient's comfort.
- The upper edge of the image detector should be positioned 3–4 cm above the spinous process of C7.

Direction and Location of the X-ray Beam

- The collimated vertical beam should be at right angles to the long axis of the thoracic vertebrae. This may (rarely) require a caudal angulation.
- The collimated beam is centred to a point 5 cm anterior to the spinous process of T6/T7. This is usually found just below the inferior angle of the scapula (assuming the arms are raised), which is easily palpable.

Essential Image Characteristics (Fig. 2.82b)

- The upper two or three vertebrae may not be demonstrated due to the superimposition of the shoulders.
- Look for the absence of a rib on L1 at the lower border of the image. This will ensure that T12 has been included within the field.
- The posterior ribs should be superimposed, thus indicating that the patient was not rotated too far forwards or backwards.

Expected DRL: DAP 1.5 Gy·cm², ESD 7 mGy

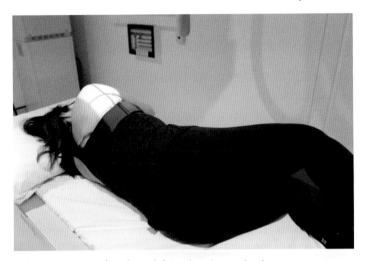

Fig. 2.82a Positioning for a lateral thoracic spine projection.

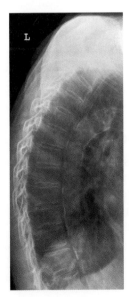

Fig. 2.82b Example of a normal lateral thoracic spine radiograph.

THUMB – ANTERO-POSTERIOR

Position of Patient and Image Receptor (Figs. 2.83a,b)

- The patient is seated facing away from the table with the arm extended backwards and medially rotated at the shoulder.
- The hand may be slightly rotated to ensure that the second, third and fourth metacarpals are not superimposed on the base of the first metacarpal.
- The patient leans forward, lowering the shoulder so that the first metacarpal is parallel to the table top.
- The detector is placed under the wrist and thumb and oriented to the long axis of the metacarpal.
- An alternative (erect) method can be used with the patient standing with the back of the hand to a vertical wall detector. The hand is internally rotated until the thumb is in a true antero-posterior position, with the first metacarpal and phalanges parallel to the detector.

Direction and Location of the X-ray Beam

- The collimated vertical beam (horizontal beam for the erect thumb method) is centred over the first metacarpo-phalangeal joint.

Essential Image Characteristics (Fig. 2.83c)

- Where there is a possibility of injury to the base of the first metacarpal, the carpo-metacarpal joint must be included on the image.

Additional Considerations

- The image should include the tip of the thumb, the distal third of the metacarpal bone and the first metacarpo-phalangeal joint and trapezium.

Notes

- A further alternative method is the postero-anterior projection, which can be used if an antero-posterior method cannot be obtained (for example in a cast). However, this method increases object-to-detector distance and hence, potentially, lack of sharpness, but it is sometimes easier and less painful for the patient.

Expected DRL: ESD 0.064 mGy

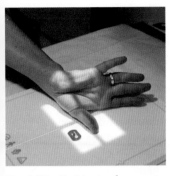 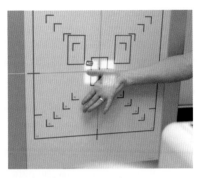

Fig. 2.83a Positioning for an antero-posterior thumb projection – sitting.

Fig. 2.83b Positioning for an antero-posterior thumb projection – standing.

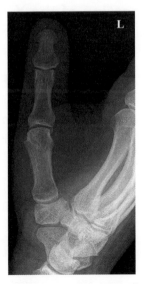

Fig. 2.83c Example of an antero-posterior thumb radiograph.

THUMB – LATERAL

Position of Patient and Image Receptor (Figs. 2.84a,b)

- The patient is seated alongside the table with the arm abducted, the elbow flexed and the anterior aspect of the forearm resting on the table.
- The thumb is flexed slightly, and the palm of the hand is placed on the image detector.
- The palm of the hand is raised slightly with the fingers partially flexed and supported on a non-opaque pad, such that the lateral aspect of the thumb is in contact with the image detector.
- Alternatively, this projection could be obtained in the erect position, using the vertical/wall detector. The patient faces the detector and stands to the side, with the palm of the hand placed on the detector and the fingers bent, to bring the thumb into a true lateral position.

Direction and Location of the X-ray Beam

- The collimated vertical beam (or horizontal beam for the erect method) is centred over the first metacarpo-phalangeal joint.

Essential Image Characteristics (Fig. 2.84c)

- Where there is a possibility of injury to the base of the first meta-carpal, the carpo-metacarpal joint must be included on the image.
- The image should include the tip of the thumb and the distal third of the metacarpal bone.

Notes

- It is common practice to obtain two projections, a lateral and an antero-posterior.
- In the case of a suspected foreign body in the thenar eminence, a postero-anterior projection is used to maintain the relationship with adjacent structures.

Expected DRL: ESD 0.064 mGy

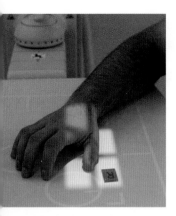

Fig. 2.84a Positioning for a lateral thumb projection – sitting.

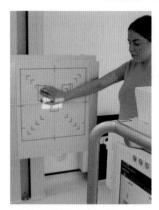

Fig. 2.84b Positioning for a lateral thumb projection – standing.

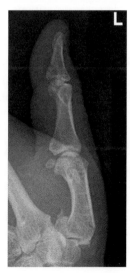

Fig. 2.84c Example of a lateral thumb radiograph.

TIBIA AND FIBULA
– ANTERO-POSTERIOR

Position of Patient and Image Receptor (Fig. 2.85a)

- The detector chosen should be large enough to accommodate the entire length of the tibia and fibula. This may require the leg to be positioned diagonally across the detector to ensure the knee joint and ankle mortise are visualised on the image.
- The patient is either supine or seated on the X-ray table or trolley, with both legs extended.
- The ankle is held in dorsiflexion and the limb is rotated medially until the medial and lateral malleoli are equidistant from the detector.
- The lower edge of the detector is positioned just below the plantar aspect of the heel.

Direction and Location of the X-ray Beam

- The collimated vertical beam is centred to the mid-shaft of the tibia with the central ray at right angles to both the long axis of the tibia and an imaginary line joining the malleoli.

Essential Image Characteristics (Figs. 2.85b,c)

- The knee and ankle joints must be included, since the proximal end of the fibula may also be fractured when there is a fracture of the distal fibula or tibia or widening of the mortise joint (Maisonneuve fracture). If a fracture of either of the tibia or fibula is seen, with overlap or shortening, then the entire length of both bones must be demonstrated (because of the bony ring rule).

Expected DRL: ESD 0.15 mGy

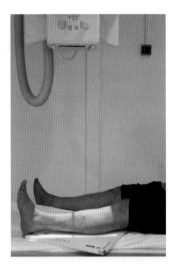

Fig. 2.85a Positioning for an antero-posterior projection of tibia and fibula.

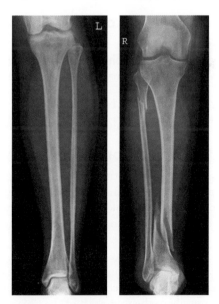

Fig. 2.85b,c Examples of antero-posterior tibia and fibula radiographs. Image (c) demonstrates proximal fibular and distal tibial fractures (bony ring rule).

Position of Patient and Image Receptor (Fig. 2.86a)

■ From the supine or seated position, the patient rotates onto the affected side.
■ The leg is rotated further until the malleoli are superimposed vertically.
■ The tibia should be parallel to the image detector.
■ A pad may be placed under the knee for support.
■ The lower edge of the detector is positioned just below the plantar aspect of the heel.
■ The detector chosen should be large enough to accommodate the entire length of the tibia and fibula. This may require the leg to be positioned diagonally across the detector to ensure the knee joint and ankle joint are included.

Direction and Location of the X-ray Beam

■ The collimated vertical beam is centred to the mid-shaft of the tibia, with the central ray at right angles to the long axis of the tibia and parallel to an imaginary line joining the malleoli.

Essential Image Characteristics (Figs. 2.86b,c)

■ The knee and ankle joints should be included on the image.

Additional Considerations

■ If it is impossible to include both joints on one image, then two images should be exposed separately, one to include the ankle and the other to include the knee. Both images should include the middle third of the lower leg, so the general alignment of the bones may be seen.
■ If it is impossible for the patient to rotate on to the affected side, then an adapted technique should be used with the detector supported vertically against the medial side of the leg and the beam directed horizontally to the mid-shaft of the tibia.

Expected DRL: ESD 0.16 mGy

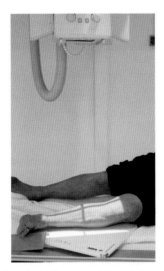

Fig. 2.86a Positioning for a lateral tibia and fibula projection.

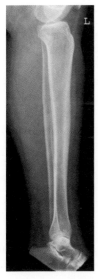

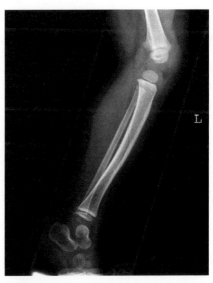

Fig. 2.86b Example of a normal tibia and fibula radiograph.

Fig. 2.86c Radiograph of a paediatric tibia and fibula, showing a spiral 'toddlers' fracture.

TOE – HALLUX – LATERAL

Position of Patient and Image Receptor (Fig. 2.87a)

- From the dorsi-plantar position, the foot is rotated medially until the medial aspect of the hallux is in contact with the image detector.
- A bandage is placed around the remaining toes (provided no injury is suspected) and they are gently pulled forwards by the patient to clear the hallux.
- Alternatively, they may be pulled backwards. This shows the meta-tarso-phalangial joint more clearly.

Direction and Location of the X-ray Beam

- The collimated vertical central beam is directed over the first met-atarso-phalangial joint.

Essential Image Characteristics (Fig. 2.87b)

- The distal and proximal phalanges, together with the distal two thirds of the first metatarsal, should be demonstrated.
- The first metatarso-phalangeal joint and inter-phalangeal should be seen clearly, with superimposition of the condyles of the head of the proximal phalanx.
- The use of this projection is important for hyper-flexion (stubbing) injuries, as an undisplaced avulsion fracture of the distal phalanx of the great toe can be missed on dorsi-plantar and dorsi-plantar oblique projections. It is important that the second to fifth toes are distracted sufficiently, to prevent superimposition of the remaining toes on the base of the proximal phalanx.

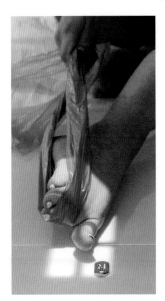

Fig. 2.87a Positioning for a lateral projection of the hallux.

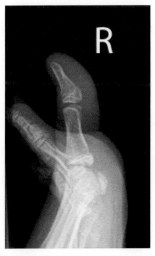

Fig. 2.87b Example of a lateral hallux radiograph.

TOES – DORSI-PLANTAR

Position of Patient and Image Receptor (Fig. 2.88a)

- The patient is seated on the X-ray table, supported if necessary, with hips and knees flexed. Alternatively, the patient is sat in a chair, with the foot placed on the wall detector placed in a horizontal position.
- The plantar aspect of the affected foot is placed on the detector. The detector may be raised by 15 degrees, using a pad or by angling the detector slightly if the wall detector is used.

Direction and Location of the X-ray Beam

- The collimated vertical central beam is directed over the third metatarso-phalangeal joint, perpendicular to the image detector if all the toes are to be imaged.
- For single toes, the vertical ray is centred over the metatarso-phalangeal joint of the individual toe and collimated to include the toe either side.

Essential Image Characteristics (Fig. 2.88b)

- The image should demonstrate the full area of interest, including the distal phalanges and proximal metatarsal region.
- A uniform radiographic contrast across the area of interest is desirable.

Additional Considerations

- It is common practice to obtain two projections, a dorsi-plantar and a dorsi-plantar oblique.
- True lateral projections of the toes are generally not requested, except in the case of the big toe, where dorsi-plantar and lateral projections are the accepted standard. True lateral projections of the big toe in paediatrics should be attempted to allow adequate evaluation of the growth plate and any Salter–Harris-type fractures, which may not be as obvious on an oblique projection.

Expected DRL: ESD 0.076 mGy

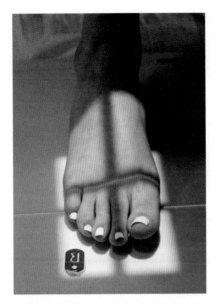

Fig. 2.88a Positioning for a dorsi-plantar toes projection.

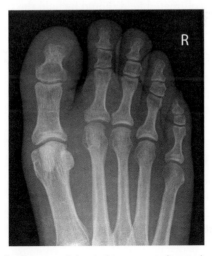

Fig. 2.88b Example of a normal dorsi-plantar toe radiograph.

TOES – SECOND TO FIFTH – DORSI-PLANTAR OBLIQUE

Position of Patient and Image Receptor (Fig. 2.89a)

- From the basic dorsi-plantar position, the affected limb is allowed to lean medially to bring the plantar surface of the foot approximately 45 degrees to the detector.
- A 45-degree non-opaque pad may be placed under the lateral side of the foot for support, with the opposite leg acting as a support.

Direction and Location of the X-ray Beam

- The collimated vertical central beam is centred over the third metatarso-phalangeal joint if all the toes are to be imaged and angled sufficiently to allow the central ray to pass through the third metatarso-phalangeal joint.
- For single toes, the vertical ray is centred over the metatarso-phalangeal joint of the individual toe, perpendicular to the detector. The collimated field should include the toe(s) adjacent to the toe in question.

Essential Image Characteristics (Fig. 2.89b)

- The image should demonstrate the full area of interest, including the distal phalanges and proximal metatarsal region.
- A uniform radiographic contrast across the area of interest is desirable.

Additional Considerations

- Ensure the foot is not over-rotated medially, which may result in toes overlapping each other.

Expected DRL: ESD 0.076 mGy

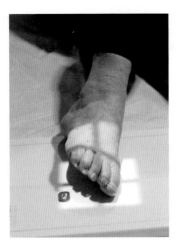

Fig. 2.89a Positioning for a dorsi-plantar oblique toe projection.

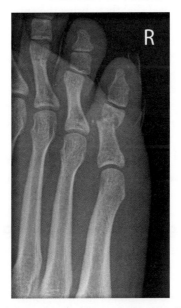

Fig. 2.89b Collimated dorsi-plantar oblique image of the fifth toe, showing an oblique displaced fracture of the 5th proximal phalanx.

WRIST – POSTERO-ANTERIOR

Position of Patient and Image Receptor (Fig. 2.90a

- The patient is seated alongside the X-ray table, or alternatively against a wall detector (grid removed) placed in a horizontal position, with the affected side nearest to the table.
- The elbow joint is flexed to 90 degrees and the arm is abducted, such that the anterior aspect of the forearm and the palm of the hand rest on the image detector.
- If the mobility of the patient permits, the shoulder joint should be at the same height as the forearm.
- The wrist joint is placed central to the image detector and adjusted to include the lower part of the radius and ulna and the proximal two thirds of the metacarpals.
- The fingers are flexed slightly to bring the anterior aspect of the wrist into contact with the image detector.
- Where possible, mild ulnar deviation of the wrist should be attempted, especially for trauma wrists, to allow adequate visualisation of the scaphoid.
- The wrist joint is adjusted to ensure that the radial and ulnar styloid processes are equidistant from the image detector.
- The forearm may be immobilised using a sandbag.

Direction and Location of the X-ray Beam

- The collimated vertical beam is centred to a point midway between the radial and ulnar styloid processes.

Essential Image Characteristics (Fig. 2.90b)

- The image should demonstrate the proximal two thirds of the metacarpals, the carpal bones and the distal third of the radius and ulna.
- There should be no rotation of the wrist joint.

Expected DRL: ESD 0.072 mGy

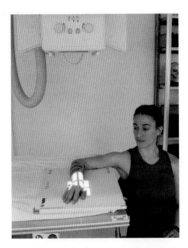

Fig. 2.90a Positioning for a postero-anterior wrist projection.

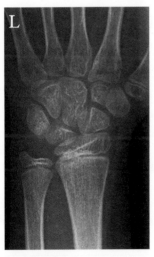

Fig. 2.90b Example of a normal paediatric postero-anterior wrist radiograph.

WRIST – LATERAL

Position of Patient and Image Receptor (Fig. 2.91a)

- The patient is seated alongside the X-ray table, or wall detector (grid removed) with the detector in the horizontal position, with the affected side nearest to the image detector.
- The elbow joint is extended to bring the medial aspect of the forearm, wrist and hand into contact with the image detector.
- The wrist joint is positioned to include the lower part of the radius and ulna and the proximal two thirds of the metacarpals on the image detector.
- The hand is rotated externally slightly further to ensure that the radial and styloid processes are superimposed.
- The forearm may be immobilised using a sandbag.

Direction and Location of the X-ray Beam

- The collimated vertical beam is centred over the styloid process of the radius.

Essential Image Characteristics (Fig. 2.91b)

- The image should demonstrate the proximal two thirds of the metacarpals, the carpal bones and the distal third of the radius and ulna.
- There should be no rotation of the wrist joint.

Notes

- If the elbow is extended rather than at right angles it is often easier to rotate the wrist into a lateral position.

Expected DRL: ESD 0.082 mGy

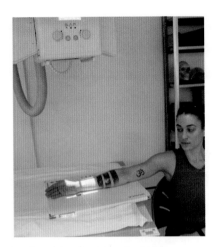

Fig. 2.91a Positioning for a lateral wrist projection.

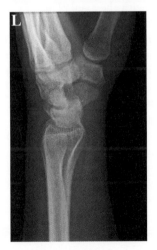

Fig. 2.91b Example of a lateral wrist radiograph.

ZYGOMATIC ARCHES – INFERO-SUPERIOR

This projection is essentially a modified submento-vertical projection to show both arches. However, a single projection called a 'jug handle' projection may be taken of the zygomatic arch in question, which is shown in profile.

Position of Patient and Image Receptor (Figs. 2.92a,b)

- The patient lies supine with one or two pillows under the shoulders to allow the neck to be fully extended.
- A detector is placed against the vertex of the skull such that its long axis is parallel with the axial plane of the body. The patient's head should be carefully supported in this position.
- The flexion of the neck is now adjusted to bring the long axis of the zygomatic arches parallel to the image detector.
- The head is now tilted 5–10 degrees away from the side under examination. This allows the zygomatic arch under examination to be projected onto the image receptor without superimposition of the skull vault or facial bones.
- Alternatively, if the patient can tolerate this position, the patient sits facing the X-ray tube a short distance away from the vertical detector/Bucky. The neck is hyperextended to allow the head to fall back until the vertex of the skull makes contact with the centre of the vertical detector.

Direction and Location of the X-ray Beam

- The central ray should be perpendicular to the detector and in the midline showing both arches. For an individual arch the beam is directed along the axis of the zygomatic arch with the centring point located such that the central ray passes through the space between the midpoint of the zygomatic arch and the lateral border of the facial bones. Close collimation should be applied to reduce scatter and to avoid irradiating the eyes.

Essential Image Characteristics (Fig. 2.92c)

The zygomatic arch injured should be fully demonstrated clear of the cranium.

Additional Considerations

A depressed fracture of the zygoma can be missed clinically due to soft tissue swelling, making the bony defect less obvious. Radiography has an important role in ensuring that potentially disfiguring depression of the cheekbones is not overlooked.

The grid is removed if using the vertical detector/Bucky method.

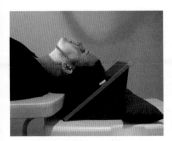
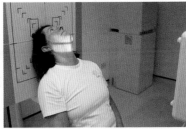

Figs. 2.92a,b Positioning for zygomatic arch projections.

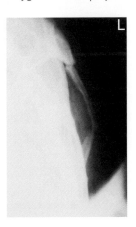

Fig. 2.92c Example of a zygomatic arch radiograph (localised), demonstrating a comminuted fracture.

SECTION 3
USEFUL INFORMATION FOR RADIOGRAPHIC PRACTICE

NON-IMAGING DIAGNOSTIC TESTS

The following blood tests are commonly performed as part of the diagnostic process. The results may have an impact upon the appropriateness of certain imaging procedures or raise suspicions of particular pathology. The reader should consult local departmental protocols for guidance in relation to some of these tests and their significance.

D-dimer

A test which measures the levels of products from the degradation of fibrin in blood clots. Raised D-dimer levels increase the suspicion of conditions such as pulmonary embolism and deep vein thrombosis. Low D-dimer levels can be used to exclude the possibility of these conditions and the need to perform expensive imaging tests.

INR: International Normalised Ratio

A measure of the time taken for blood to clot. A normal result would be around 1.0 but patients who are taking anticoagulant drugs may have a value of 2.0–3.5. Invasive diagnostic tests, such as angiography, may be contraindicated with patients with a high INR due to the subsequent risk of haemorrhage (see local departmental protocols for guidance).

e-GFR: Estimated Glomerular Filtration Rate

Used to measure the health of the kidneys and renal function. It takes into account variables such as age, sex and serum creatinine levels. Levels of greater than 90 mL/min/1.73 m^2 are considered normal. Levels below this value indicate impaired renal function.

ESR: Erythrocyte Sedimentation Rate

A non-specific test which measures the time taken for red blood cells to settle in a thin tube of liquid. Various diseases will affect the ability of the cells to do this and will increase the time taken for the cells to settle. Some examples of such diseases include those which cause inflammation, auto-immune diseases and cancers, including myeloma. Typical normal values for adults are between 10 and 20 mm/hour. This value varies considerably with age. Values of over 100 mm/hour would be of significant concern.

Serum Creatinine

Creatinine is a metabolic waste product which is excreted from the blood plasma by the kidneys. A raised serum creatinine indicates impaired renal function (normal levels are typically in the range of 0.6–1.2 mg/dL). Patients with raised serum creatinine may be at an increased risk from renal failure if iodinated contrast agents are administered (see local departmental protocols for guidance).

LFTs: Liver Function Tests

A group of tests which are used to assess the overall health of the liver and biliary system. Abnormal tests can give early indications of serious conditions. If the liver is diseased and the cells are damaged, various enzymes will be released into the bloodstream, for example alanine transaminase (ALT) or alkaline phosphatase (ALP). Disease may also affect the ability of the liver to produce albumin. High levels of bilirubin in the blood indicate jaundice.

PSA: Prostate-specific Antigen

This is an enzyme produced by the prostate gland which can be measured in the blood. A raised level of PSA could indicate the presence of prostate cancer although the test can be misleading. Some men with raised levels of PSA may not have cancer and those with normal levels may actually have the disease. A level of 3.0–4.0 ng/mL or below is considered normal.

CA125: Cancer Antigen 125

A blood test used to diagnose ovarian cancer. A normal value would range between 0 and 35 U/mL. A value above this would not always indicate the presence of a tumour but would certainly indicate further investigations.

hCG: Human Chorionic Gonadotropin

A hormone produced by the placenta which can be measured in the blood or urine to confirm an early pregnancy. Raised levels of hCG in the absence of pregnancy may indicate a tumour.

MEDICAL TERMINOLOGY

The following list of common prefixes and suffixes can be employed to work out the meaning of complex disease terminology encountered on requests for radiological examinations.

Prefixes

A- *or* An-	absence of or without
Adreno-	relating to the adrenal glands
Angio-	relating to blood or lymph vessels
Ante-	in front or before
Arterio-	relating to arteries
Bi-	two
Brady-	too slow
Bucc-	relating to the cheek
Burs-	relating to bursa within synovial joints
Cardi-	relating to the heart
Cebr-	relating to the brain
Cephal-	relating to the head
Cervic-	neck
Chol-	relating to the biliary system or bile
Crani-	relating to the skull
Cysto-	relating to the bladder or gall baldder
Dacro-	relating to tears and associated glands or ducts
Dacry-	relating to tears
Demi-	half
Dorsi-	back
Dys-	difficulty
Ec-	away from or not in usual position
Endo-	inside or within
Ente-	relating to the intestine
Epi-	upon
Erythro-	reddening or flushing of
Ex-	out of
Gastr-	relating to the stomach
Gingiv-	relating to the gums

Haem-	relating to the blood
Hemi-	half
Hydro-	water
Hyper-	beyond normal limits
Hypo-	below normal limits
Hystr(o)-	relating to the uterus
Idio-	relating to an individual or self
Infra-	below
Inter-	between
Intra-	within
Iso-	the same as
Lact-	milk
Laparo-	relating to the abdomen wall
Leuco-	relating to white blood cells
Lingu-	relating to the tongue
Lipo-	relating to fat
Litho-	stone formation
Lympho-	relating to the lymphatic system
Lysis-	destruction of
Macro-	large
Mammo- or Masto-	relating to the breast
Mega-	enlargement of
Myo-	muscle
Neo-	new
Nephro-	relating to the kidney
Neuro-	relating to the nervous system
Orchid-	relating to the testes
Osteo-	relating to the bones
Peri-	around
Phleb-	relating to the veins
Pneumo-	relating to the lungs
Poly-	many
Post-	after
Pyo-	relating to pus
Retro-	behind
Salpingo-	relating to the uterine tubes
Sial-	relating to the salivary glands
Spleno-	relating to the spleen

259

Spondy-	relating to the spine
Sub-	beneath
Supra-	above, upper
Syn-	together
Tachy-	too fast
Trach-	relating to the trachea
Trans-	through
Urin- *or* uro-	relating to the urinary system or urine
Vesico-	relating to the bladder

Suffixes

-aemia	disease affecting the blood
-algia	pain
-ectasis	enlargement or widening of
-ectomy	the surgical removal of
-itis	inflammation of
-oma	tumour
-oscopy	the visual examination of
-ostomy	surgical opening of
-osis	disease of
-penia	lack of
-plasty	repair or reconstruction
-rrhoea	flow

MEDICAL AND RADIOGRAPHIC ABBREVIATIONS

AAA	abdominal aortic aneurysm
ACL	anterior cruciate ligament
AE	air entry
AEC	automatic exposure control
AF	atrial fibrillation
AFP	alpha-fetoprotein
ALL	acute lymphocytic leukaemia
ALP	alkaline phosphatase
ALT	alanine transaminase
AML	acute myelogenous leukaemia
AP	antero-posterior
ARDS	acute respiratory distress syndrome
ASD	atrial septal defect
AVM	arteriovenous malformation
AXR	abdomen X-ray
BE	barium enema
BI	bony injury
BMI	body mass index
BP	blood pressure
Ca	cancer
CABG	coronary artery bypass graft
CAT	computed axial tomography
CBD	common bile duct
CN	cranial nerve
CO	complains of
COPD	chronic obstructive pulmonary disease
COVID-19	coronavirus disease 2019
CPR	cardiopulmonary resuscitation
CR	computed radiography
CSF	cerebrospinal fluid

CT	computed tomography
CTR	cardiothoracic ratio
CVA	cerebrovascular accident (stroke)
CVP	central venous pressure
CXR	chest X-ray
D&C	dilation and curettage
D&V	diarrhoea and vomiting
DAP	dose-area product
DDI	detector dose indicator
DDR	direct digital radiography
DDx	differential diagnosis
DI	deviation index
DIP	distal interphalangeal (joint)
DNA	did not attend *or* deoxyribonucleic acid
DPT	dental panoramic tomography
DR	digital radiography
DRL	diagnostic reference level
DVT	deep vein thrombosis
DX	diagnosis
DXT	deep X-ray treatment
EAM	external auditory meatus
ECG	electrocardiogram
ECT	electroconvulsive therapy
EDD	estimated date of delivery
EI	exposure index
EI_T	target exposure index
ENT	ear, nose and throat
ERCP	endoscopic retrograde cholangio-pancreatography
ESD	entrance skin dose
ESR	erythrocyte sedimentation rate
ET	endotracheal
FB	foreign body
FBC	full blood count
FH	family history
FO	fronto-occipital

FOD	focus-to-object distance
FRD	focus-to-receptor distance
FTT	failure to thrive
FUO	fever of unknown origin
GCS	Glasgow Coma Scale
GFR	glomerular filtration rate
GIT	gasterointestinal tract
GU	gastric ulcer *or* genito-urinary
Gy	Gray (unit of ionising radiation dose)
Hb	haemoglobin
HI	head injury
HIV	human immunodeficiency virus
Hx	history of
IAM	internal auditory meatus
ICRP 84	International Commission on Radiological Protection pregnancy and medical radiation guidelines
ICU	intensive care unit
ID	identification
IDDM	insulin-dependent diabetes mellitus
IDK	internal derangement of the knee
IM	intramedullary *or* intramuscular
IR(ME)R 17	Ionising Radiation (Medical Exposure) Regulations 2017 (amended 2018)
IRR17	Ionising Radiation Regulations 2017
ITU	intensive treatment unit
IVC	inferior vena cava *or* intravenous cholangiogram
IVP	intravenous pyelogram
IVU	intravenous urogram
KUB	kidneys, ureters and bladder
kV	kilovolt
LAO	left anterior oblique
LLL	left lower lobe
LOC	loss of consciousness

LP	lumbar puncture
LUL	left upper lobe
LUQ	left upper quadrant
LVF	left ventricular failure
mAs	milliamp-second
MCP	metacarpo-phalangeal
MI	myocardial infarction
MPE	medical physics expert
MRI	magnetic resonance imaging
MRSA	methicillin-resistant *Staphylococcus aureus*
MS	multiple sclerosis *or* mitral stenosis
MSP	median sagittal plane
NAD	no abnormality detected
NBI	no bony injury
NBM	nil by mouth
NFR	not for resuscitation
NFS	no fracture seen
NG	nasogastric *or* new growth
NIDDM	non-insulin-dependent diabetes mellitus
NMR	nuclear magnetic resonance
NSAID	non-steroidal anti-inflammatory drug
OA	osteoarthritis
OE	on examination
OF	occipito-frontal
OM	occipito-mental
OPG	orthopantomography
ORD	object-to-receptor distance
ORIF	open reduction and internal fixation
PA	postero-anterior
PACS	picture archiving and communication system
PE	pulmonary embolus
PID	prolapsed intervertebral disc *or* pelvic inflammatory disease
PIJ	proximal interphalangeal joint
PNS	post-nasal space

POP	plaster of Paris
PPE	protective personal equipment
PR	per (via) the rectum
PRN	as often as needed
PTCA	percutaneous transluminal coronary angioplasty
PUO	pyrexia of unknown origin
PV	per (via) the vagina
QA	quality assurance
RA	rheumatoid arthritis
RAO	right anterior oblique
RBC	red blood cell
RLL	right lower lobe
RML	right middle lobe
ROI	region of interest
RPS	radiation protection supervisor
RT	radiotherapy
RTC	road traffic collision
RUL	right upper lobe
RUQ	right upper quadrant
Rx	treatment
SAH	subarachnoid haemorrhage
SBE	subacute bacterial endocarditis
SLE	systemic lupus erythematosus
SMV	submento-vertical
SOB	shortness of breath
SOL	space-occupying lesion
STD	sexually transmitted disease
Sv	sievert (unit of radiation dose, measuring energy absorbed)
Sx	symptoms
SXR	skull X-ray
TB	tuberculosis
TFT	thyroid function test
THR	total hip replacement

TIA	transient ischaemic attack
TKR	total knee replacement
TMJ	temporo-mandibular joint
TPR	temperature, pulse and respiration
TURP	transurethral resection of prostate
Tx	treatment
U&E	urea and electrolytes
UC	ulcerative colitis
URTI	upper respiratory tract infection
US	ultrasound
UTI	urinary tract infection
VF	ventricular fibrillation
V/Q	lung perfusion/ventilation scan
VSD	ventricular septal defect
VT	ventricular tachycardia
WBC	white blood cell count
YO	years old
0	not present
+	present
++	present significantly
+++	present substantially
↑ / ↓	increase/decrease
#	fracture
1/7	1 day
2/52	two weeks
3/12	three months

INDEX